THE HUMAN HEART
A Basic Guide
to Heart Disease

Second Edition

BRENDAN PHIBBS, MD

Professor of Clinical Medicine, Section of Cardiology,
University of Arizona College of Medicine
Tucson, Arizona

Illustrations by
Christopher Wikoff

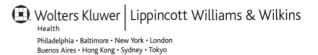

Wolters Kluwer | Lippincott Williams & Wilkins
Health

Philadelphia · Baltimore · New York · London
Buenos Aires · Hong Kong · Sydney · Tokyo

Acquisitions Editor: Fran DeStefano
Developmental Editor: Fran Murphy
Managing Editor: Julia Seto
Project Manager: Nicole Walz
Manufacturing Coordinator: Kathleen Brown
Marketing Manager: Angela Panetta
Art Director: Risa Clow
Cover Designer: Joseph DePinho
Production Service: GGS Book Services
Printer: Edwards Brothers

Printed in the USA

Library of Congress Cataloging-in-Publication Data

Phibbs, Brendan.
        The human heart : a basic guide to heart disease / Brendan Phibbs; illustrations by Christopher Wikoff. — 2nd ed.
            p. ; cm.
        Includes bibliographical references and index.
        ISBN-13: 978-0-7817-6777-4 (pbk.)
        ISBN-10: 0-7817-6777-6 (pbk.)
        1. Heart—Diseases.   2. Heart—Pathophysiology.   3. Heart—Physiology   I. Title.
        [DNLM: 1. Heart Diseases.   2. Heart—Physiology.   WG 210 P543h 2007]
    RC681. P529 2007
    616.1' 2—dc22

To purchase additional copies of this book, call our customer service department at **(800) 638-3030** or fax orders to **(301) 223-2320.** International customers should call **(301) 223-2300.**

Visit Lippincott Williams & Wilkins on the Internet: at LWW.com. Lippincott Williams & Wilkins customer service representatives are available from 8:30 am to 6 pm, EST.

10 9 8 7 6 5 4 3 2 1

THE HUMAN HEART

A Basic Guide
to Heart Disease

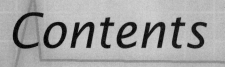

Contents

Preface   vii

CHAPTER 1   Structure and Function of the Normal Heart   1

CHAPTER 2   Valves of the Heart   6

CHAPTER 3   Pumping Action of the Heart   9

CHAPTER 4   Blood Supply of the Heart   11

CHAPTER 5   The Functioning Normal Heart   13

CHAPTER 6   Heart Failure   21

CHAPTER 7   Hypertensive Heart Disease   25

CHAPTER 8   Coronary Artery Disease   41

CHAPTER 9   The Heart Valves   65

CHAPTER 10   The Autonomic or Automatic Nervous System   77

CHAPTER 11   The Electrocardiogram   80

CHAPTER 12   Cardiac Arrhythmias   90

CHAPTER 13   Congenital Heart Disease   120

CHAPTER 14   Rheumatic Heart Disease   132

CHAPTER 15   Pregnancy and Heart Disease   138

CHAPTER 16   Pulmonary Heart Disease   143

CHAPTER 17   Imaginary Heart Disease   147

CHAPTER 18   To Pace or Not to Pace   150

CHAPTER 19   Medical Treatment of Heart Failure   156

CHAPTER 20   Catheterization of the Heart and Coronary Arteriography   164

CHAPTER 21   Cardiac Surgery   168

CHAPTER 22   Heart Attack   178

CHAPTER 23   Measuring the Efficiency of the Heart   188

CHAPTER 24   Special Diagnostic Procedures   190

REVIEW TEST   195

ANSWERS   201

APPENDIX Notes for Coronary Intensive Units   207

INDEX   220

Preface

*T*his book began as a handbook for cardiac patients. It's now been used by coronary-intensive-care nurses, paramedics, emergency-room personnel, family practitioners, hospitalists, pharmaceutical companies, and others.

"It can't be that simple!"
One of my medical students blurted that out after I explained bundle-branch block. Yes, I told him, it is. It's a simple phenomenon, easily diagnosed: the only thing complicated about it is the murky, confused language some people use to describe it.

If you can read ordinary, non-technical basic English, you can understood what's in this book. I guarantee it.

Most of the facts about medicine can be stated in clear, easily understood language if the writer will only make the effort to do so.

This is the sixth edition (second edition published by Lippincott Williams & Wilkins) of a book that's been in use for about forty years: requests for it have come from as far away as the Republic of Mauritius, so it seems to be filling a large niche. That niche has been created by medical gibberish. For example: On a chart a nurse noted that the patient "ambulated, became diaphoretic, and expired." I wrote beneath that the patient in fact "walked, sweated, and died."

Mobitz-II heart block is a dangerous abnormality that threatens sudden death and automatically calls for a pacemaker. A shocking number of physicians (and some cardologists) don't know how to diagnose it. If you read Chapter 12, you'll absolutely know how to recognize it—and that will put you in the upper one or two percent of the medical world.

This book is revised because in the world of medicine new information comes streaming like Niagara Falls. For example, my colleagues here at the University of Arizona have absolutely revolutionized the treatment of cardiac arrest, and their findings are saving thousands of lives in many parts of the U.S. and abroad. When someone collapses, pulseless, you compress the heart much faster than we used to and you *don't* start mouth-to-mouth breathing. It turns out that the time wasted in mouth-to-mouth breathing was lethal! Please read about this new revolutionary treatment.

Coronary artery disease can be treated by medical management, angioplasty or bypass surgery. In many patients, angioplasty and bypass surgery only relieve pain—*they don't prolong life*. We now know pretty well which kinds of coronary disease fall into the "relieve pain" or "prolong life" categories, and the patient should have this information to help in what may be a life or death decision.

More than ever, care of cardiovascular disease involves a team that starts with the patient and family members and extends to ambulance and emergency-room personnel, coronary-intensive care nurses, interns, residents, and attending physicians. A weak link anywhere can be a disaster.

Ignorance is not bliss—it's frequently fatal. *Mehr licht!* said Goethe, more light! Be informed!

Brendan Phibbs, MD

CHAPTER 1

Structure and Function of the Normal Heart

Before you begin to learn about heart disease, you must learn how the normal heart is constructed and how it functions. This is easier than you might think, because the heart is a surprisingly simple organ. An hour's easy reading will give you all the information you need to begin.

THE CHAMBERS OF THE HEART AND THEIR CONNECTIONS

The heart is a hollow organ divided into four chambers, two on the top and two on the bottom (Fig. 1–1). Study this simple diagram until you know it as well as your own name: it's basic to everything else in the book.

The top two chambers are thin-walled structures that act primarily as holding chambers for the blood. They are called **atria**. This is the plural of the Latin word *atrium*, meaning "anteroom" or "porch," and, in fact, these chambers do act as entryways to the great chambers below. The **ventricles** are large, thick-walled chambers that do the real work of pumping the blood. (This name comes from the Latin *ventriculum*, meaning a "cavity" or "pouch.")

Look again at Figure 1–1 and note the wall, or septum, that divides the left atrium from the right atrium and the left ventricle from the right ventricle. This wall of tissue is much like the septum in your nose that separates the two nostrils. The important thing to remember about the heart's septum is that it is absolutely watertight, or, more properly, "bloodtight." Normally, no blood can pass through this septum from one side to the other. (It took the human race about 4,000 years to discover this simple fact. The ancient Greeks and Romans were convinced that blood somehow oozed through the septum from one side to the other. It doesn't.)

Physicians commonly refer to the right atrium and right ventricle together as the **right heart** and to the left atrium and left ventricle as the **left heart.**

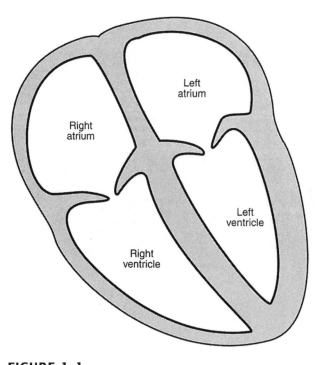

FIGURE 1–1
The chambers of the heart.

THE MOTION OF THE BLOOD THROUGH THE HEART

The function of the heart can be described as a simple pump that forces blood forward by squeezing, in exactly the way that a bulb syringe forces out fluid when it's compressed.

The alert reader will at once ask, "If the blood doesn't flow from one side of the heart to the other through the septum, how does it ever move forward?" The answer to that question eluded philosophers and scientists until the English medical doctor William Harvey, in the early seventeenth century, discovered the simple circuit that is the basis of all modern cardiology.

The blood moves from the right heart to the left heart by way of the lungs. In other words, the right heart pulls the blood out of the veins and pumps it into the lungs. The left heart pulls the blood out of the lungs and pumps it on to the body.

(The outraged squalling of Harvey's contemporaries and the hoots of disbelief that greeted this profound truth are amusing to contemplate; they are also a little frightening.) Thus the heart and lungs together form a machine that takes oxygen out of the air, dissolves it in the blood, and pumps it to the tissues of the body.

BACK TO STRUCTURE: HOW ARE THE HEART AND LUNGS CONNECTED?

The blood that has completed its course through the tissues of the body flows back to the heart through the veins. The veins come together, growing larger, like streams combining into a river, until they end in two great veins that empty into the top and bottom

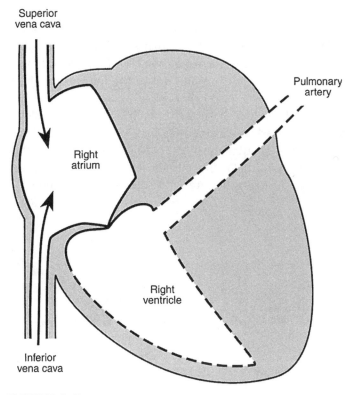

FIGURE 1–2
Blood entering the right atrium.

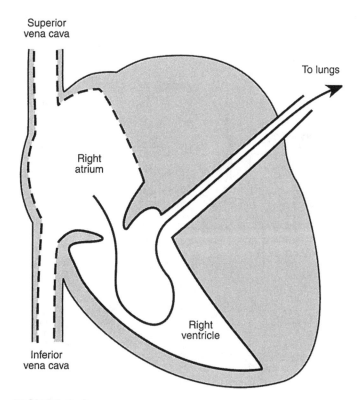

FIGURE 1–3
Blood flowing from the right ventricle.

of the right atrium. The word *cava* in Latin refers to something large or cavelike; hence the vein that empties into the top of the right atrium is called the **superior vena cava**, or, literally, "large top vein." The great vein that empties into the bottom of the right atrium is logically called the **inferior vena cava** (Fig. 1–2). Blood flows from the right atrium down into the right ventricle and out to the lungs through the **pulmonary artery** (Fig. 1–3).

Within the lungs, the pulmonary artery branches into ever smaller arteries until it ends in a mass of **capillaries**—tiny vessels just wide enough to let one blood cell through at a time (Fig. 1–4). After the blood has been oxygenated it flows back to the heart through the four veins that empty into the left atrium (Fig. 1–5). Since these veins flow from the lungs to the heart they are called the **pulmonary veins.**

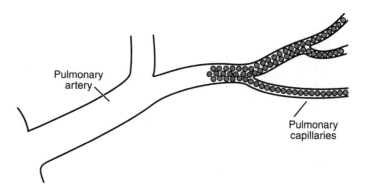

FIGURE 1–4
Blood flowing to the lungs through the pulmonary artery.

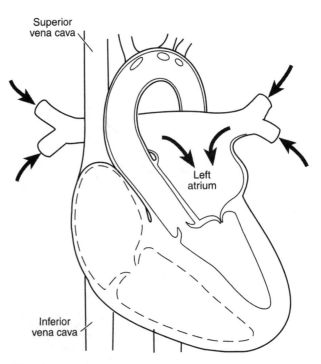

FIGURE 1–5
Blood returning from the lungs to the left atrium.

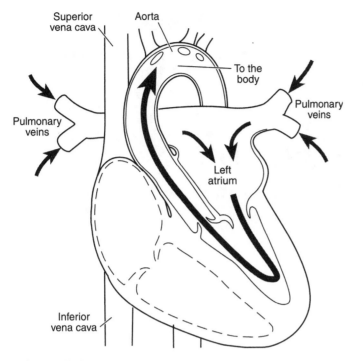

FIGURE 1–6
After flowing to the left ventricle, blood flows out through the
aorta to the body.

From the left atrium, blood flows down into the left ventricle and then out the
aorta to the body (Fig. 1–6).

You must be thoroughly familiar with this circuit and with the names and function
of the great vessels of the heart and lungs. The **great vessels of the heart** is the term
used to include both arteries and veins.

Note: The great vessels of the heart are as follows:

* *The* superior and inferior vena cavae, *that empty all the blood from the body into
  the right atrium.*
* *The* pulmonary artery, *which carries blood from the right ventricle to the lungs.*
* *The* pulmonary veins, *which carry oxygenated blood from the lungs to the left
  atrium.*
* *The* aorta, *or great artery, which carries the oxygenated blood out of the left
  ventricle to the body.*

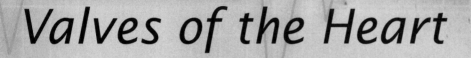

CHAPTER 2

Valves of the Heart

VALVE STRUCTURE AND FUNCTION

Like any pump, the heart has valves to keep the blood flowing in the right direction. Proper function of these small flaps of tissue spells the difference between good health and sickness, and often between life and death.

Almost everyone is familiar with the word *valve*. Very few people, however, really know what a valve is or what it does. Imagine pumping water through a pipe with a farm pump. To keep the water from flowing back toward the pump between strokes, you could place a valve in the pipe leading out of the pump. The simplest kind of valve would consist of two semicircular flaps hinged to open only one way—forward with the flow of water. These flaps would close the pipe completely when they swung shut. When the water flowed forward from the pump, the flaps of the valve would swing open allowing the water to pass. Between strokes the valves would snap shut if any water attempted to flow back toward the pump (Fig. 2–1).

Note: The heart is equipped with four sets of valves that function on this simple principle:

- *tricuspid valve*
- *mitral valve*
- *pulmonic valve*
- *aortic valve*

The valves between the atria and ventricles are called the **atrioventricular (AV) valves**. The AV valve leading into the right ventricle has three flaps and is called the **tricuspid valve** (a cusp is a valve flap or leaflet).

The AV valve that swings into the left ventricle is called the **mitral valve**. (It has two cusps and therefore looks something like a bishop's miter.)

Each of the outlet valves from the ventricles has three cusps. The valve at the entry to the pulmonary artery is called the **pulmonic valve**. The valve at the entry to the aorta is called the **aortic valve**.

As stated, an AV valve is located between each atrium and ventricle (Fig. 2–2). This valve opens downward into the ventricle. During diastole, or relaxation, the valves swing

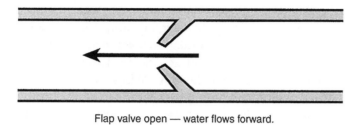

Flap valve open — water flows forward.

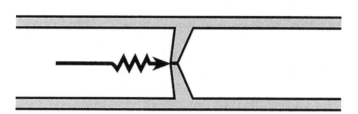

Flap valve shut — water cannot flow back.

FIGURE 2–1
How a watertight valve functions.

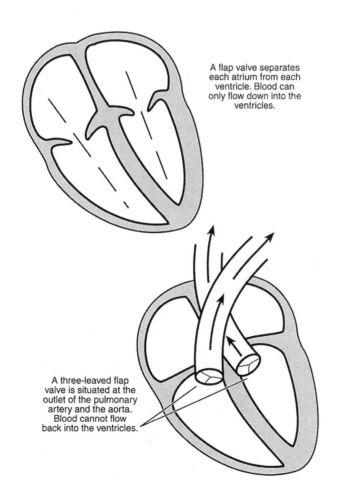

A flap valve separates each atrium from each ventricle. Blood can only flow down into the ventricles.

A three-leaved flap valve is situated at the outlet of the pulmonary artery and the aorta. Blood cannot flow back into the ventricles.

FIGURE 2–2
Valves of the heart.

open, allowing the blood to flow down into the ventricles. When the ventricles contract, these valves snap shut, preventing any blood from flowing back up into the atria.

A valve is also located at the outlet from each ventricle into the great vessel leaving the chamber. When the ventricles contract, these valves are forced open; the blood rushes into the pulmonary artery and the aorta. When the ventricles relax, the valves close, shutting off any backward flow into the ventricles.

If the heart is to function efficiently, these valves must be absolutely watertight, or more properly, bloodtight. Further, they must open freely and widely to let the blood flow forward with the pumping action of the heart. If the valves leak or if they are partly closed by adhesions or hardening, the heart works against a mechanical load, often an impossible and fatal load, as will be discussed in later chapters.

LAYERS OF THE HEART

The heart does not simply hang freely in the chest cavity; around it is a loose protective sack of tissue called the **pericardium**. The heart lies inside this sack, which is loose enough to permit the heart to beat easily. Picture a turnip held in a heavy, double thickness plastic bag. This is about the way the heart looks inside the pericardium (Fig. 2–3).

If the pericardium is cut open, the surface of the heart itself appears shiny and reddish in color. You can actually peel away a thin, shiny membrane from the outer surface of the heart. This membrane is called the **epicardium**. The mass of the heart is muscle; under the epicardium is a thick layer of muscle called the **myocardium**, which forms the actual working part of the heart. The myocardium is thickest in the left ventricle; it is thinnest in the atria. The cells in the myocardium are a specialized type of muscle, different from anything else in the body.

The inside of the heart, or cavity, is lined with another smooth, shiny membrane much like the inside surface of the cheek. This thin membrane, called the **endocardium**, covers the inside of the chambers of the heart. It also covers the heart valves and the small muscles associated with the opening and closing of these valves.

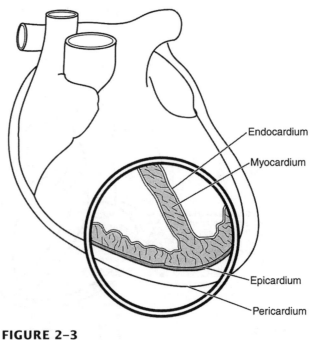

FIGURE 2–3
Layers of the heart.

CHAPTER 3

Pumping Action of the Heart

BLOOD FLOW THROUGH THE HEART

Blood is pumped through the chambers of the heart and out through the great vessels by a simple squeezing action of the heart chambers. You have probably seen a bulb syringe with a glass nozzle like the one pictured in Figure 3–1. Suppose it is full of water. If you squeeze forcefully, expelling the water, you would be imitating the contraction of a heart chamber. This is called **systole** (sis-toe-lee). After the syringe had been emptied, imagine that you placed the nozzle in a container of water and let the bulb expand so that it filled. This is what a heart chamber does when it relaxes and fills with blood. The movement is called **diastole** (die-as-toe-lee). You can picture the process by holding your left hand over your right, fists clenched. If your left hand represents the atria, your right hand will represent the ventricles. Now clench your left fist (the atria) while opening your right fist (the ventricles). This is what happens during atrial systole when the atria are pumping blood down into the ventricles. Next, open your left fist and clench your right. This is what happens during ventricular systole when the ventricles are pumping blood out into the two great arteries and the atria are refilling. By alternately opening and clenching your two fists you can similate the coordinated beat of the heart.

Note: The cycle of a heartbeat, in other words, goes through these stages:

- *Atrial systole: The atria contract, forcing the blood down into the ventricles.*
- *Ventricular systole: The ventricles contract, forcing the blood out the pulmonary artery and aorta.*
- *Atrial diastole: This starts during ventricular systole as the atria begin refilling with blood from the great veins.*
- *Ventricular diastole: This takes place during atrial systole as blood from the atria fills the ventricles.*

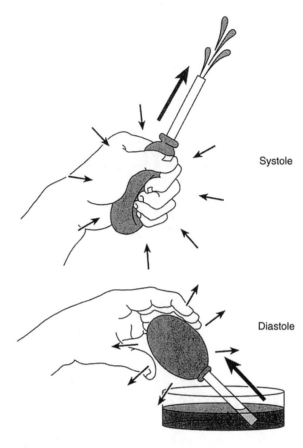

Systole

Diastole

FIGURE 3–1
Expelling liquid from a bulb syringe is similar to the
pumping action of the heart.

The rhythmic contraction and relaxation of the ventricles does the work of pumping the blood: atrial contraction is much less important and, in fact, many patients live for years without any pumping action from the atria. If the ventricles stop beating, death follows within minutes.

Blood Supply of the Heart

HEART STRUCTURE AND BLOOD SUPPLY

It seems odd that the tissues making up the heart must have their own separate blood supply. You might think that the torrent of blood rushing through the heart every minute would more than adequately meet the needs of the organ. The walls of the heart, however, consist of layers of specialized muscle. These walls are quite thick—the wall of the left ventricle is often over 1 inch thick. Since the lining of the heart is watertight, the blood cannot seep through the layers of muscle to provide the nourishment essential to these constantly working masses. Blood is carried through the muscle layers that form the heart wall by means of the two **coronary arteries**. These two small vessels branch off the aorta just after it leaves the heart and curl back across the surface of the chambers, sending twigs through the walls (Fig. 4–1).

The coronary arteries are so named because of the supposed resemblance to a crown or "corona" of the little arteries as they encircle the heart. These arteries divide into smaller and smaller branches, like all blood vessels in the body, until they become so small that only one blood cell at a time can move through them. At this point the vessels are called **capillaries**. After the blood has passed through the capillaries, and the tissues have extracted the needed oxygen, it returns by way of veins, which become larger and larger until they, like all other veins in the body, empty into the right atrium. The veins from the wall of the heart, or coronary veins, empty into the right atrium through a structure called the **coronary sinus**.

The blood supply of the tissues in the wall of the heart is not very good; thousands of people die every year because of this curious fact. Most organs and tissues of the body have a "reserve" or collateral blood supply. Each finger, for instance, has two arteries, one on each side. These arteries are connected by many cross-channels, or collateral vessels. If the artery is cut on one side, the collateral or cross-connections from the artery on the other side would probably provide sufficient blood to maintain life in the tissues of the finger. The same "safety" feature is true in most of the major areas of the body. It is not true in the wall of the heart.

The coronary arteries tend to be **end arteries**, meaning that each branch follows its own course to some area of the heart muscle with relatively few connections to

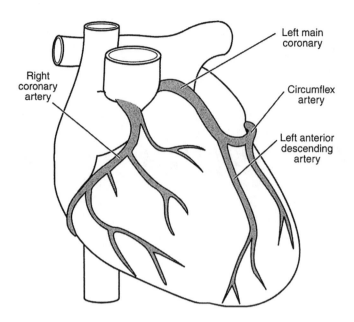

FIGURE 4–1
Coronary arteries.

other branches nearby. If one of these coronary branches is plugged by hardening or by a blood clot, the muscle that depends on it for blood will die. A form of gangrene actually sets in. (Some people's coronary arteries have many more cross-connections than others. The more of these cross-connections an individual has, the less likely he or she is to die of coronary artery disease. In 10,000 or 20,000 years the process of evolution may result in a race with a good coronary blood supply by virtue of the early death of those without it.)

The names of the chief branches of the coronary arteries are important because they will be used repeatedly in this book. Learn them now; they're very simple.

There are two main coronary arteries leading out of the aorta—the **right** and **left coronary arteries**. After about an inch, the left coronary artery divides into two principal branches. The **left anterior descending** branch comes down the front of the heart, roughly along the septum between the two ventricles. The **circumflex** branch of the left coronary artery coils around the left side and back of the heart. The right coronary artery divides into a number of branches that course through the right chambers of the heart as well as through a large part of the left ventricle.

Note: There are four coronary arteries to remember:

- *The left main coronary artery (before it divides): LMCA.*
- *The right coronary artery: RCA.*
- *The left anterior descending branch of the left main coronary artery: LAD.*
- *The circumflex branch of the left main coronary artery: LCA or LCirc.*

CHAPTER 5

The Functioning Normal Heart

COORDINATION OF THE HEARTBEAT, THE VALVES, AND THE FLOW OF BLOOD

To understand an engine, it isn't enough to learn about its parts. You have to turn on the machine and watch it function. How is the heartbeat coordinated in various chambers? What keeps the blood from going backward instead of forward? How is the heartbeat timed so that each chamber is ready to receive the inrush of blood at the right split second? Watch a sample of blood move through the heart–lung machine and see how everything is coordinated.

Systole

The ventricles contract and the pressure inside them rises. When the pressure inside the ventricles is higher than the pressure inside the atria, the atrioventricular (AV) valves are slammed shut, just as if the pressure of your hand was closing a door. In other words, the mitral and tricuspid valves are forced shut early in ventricular systole. The inrush of blood from the veins fills the atria against these closed valves.

The same rise in pressure forces the outlet valves open, so that blood can flow out of the ventricle into the pulmonary artery and the aorta. The aortic and pulmonic valves are forced open early in systole (Fig. 5–1).

Diastole

The ventricles relax and the pressure in them falls. When it falls below the pressure in the atria, the AV valves swing open and blood rushes into the ventricles. The mitral and tricuspid valves are forced open early in diastole.

The same fall in pressure drops the pressure in the ventricles below the pressure in the great vessels (the aorta and the pulmonary artery). The higher pressure in

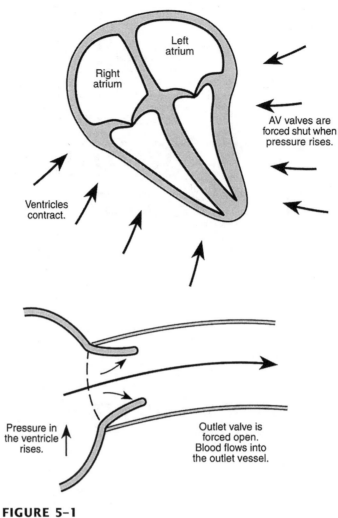

FIGURE 5–1
The events of systole.

the great vessels forces the outlet valves shut, holding the blood in the lungs and in the whole body.

The aortic and pulmonic valves are forced shut early in diastole (Fig. 5–2).

THE ELECTRIC CIRCUIT THAT DRIVES THE HEART

The muscles that move your body can't function by themselves: they can only contract when they are stimulated by a nerve impulse. This impulse is actually a wave of electric energy that starts in the brain and travels down a nerve to the muscles involved in a particular motion. If the nerve is cut or if the brain tissue is destroyed, the muscles will be paralyzed (Fig. 5–3).

The heart is different. It has its own self-contained "nerve" system to stimulate it to beat. The cells that make up this system are really heart muscle cells, specially adapted, but they function as nerve cells.

The electric energy that stimulates the heart muscle begins in a small bundle of tissue less than 0.5 inch long located near the top of the right atrium. This very important

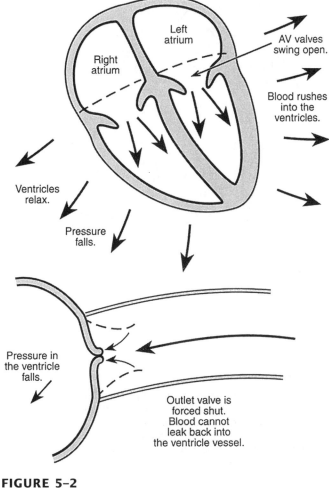

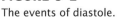

FIGURE 5–2
The events of diastole.

structure is called the **sinoatrial node,** often abbreviated as the **SA node.** The sinoatrial node is the source of the electric energy that makes the heart beat: it builds up a definite potential and then discharges, sending a wave of electric energy spreading across the atria, like a ripple across a pond. When muscle is stimulated by an electric impulse, it contracts (you probably remember the way your hand jerked when you touched a live light socket as a child). The cells of the atrial walls transmit the activating impulse from cell to cell. This meshwork of cells is called the **atrial syncytium** (Fig. 5–4).

There is a bundle of conducting tissue leading out of the atria, like a small canal leading out of a pond. This bundle connects the atria and the ventricles and is logically named the **atrioventricular** or **AV node.** The cells in the atrioventricular node are specialized: they conduct the activating current of the heart just as an electric wire might conduct current from a battery to a lightbulb. The lower end of the AV node is called the bundle of His—it's a little different in structure from the upper part. The bottom of the bundle of His divides into two branches, one to each ventricle. Logically, these are called the **left** and **right bundle branches.** The bundle branches divide into progressively smaller twigs, exactly like the branches of a tree. They end in small fibers called the **Purkinje fibers.** These tiny elements actually transmit the electric charge to the heart muscle (Fig. 5–5).

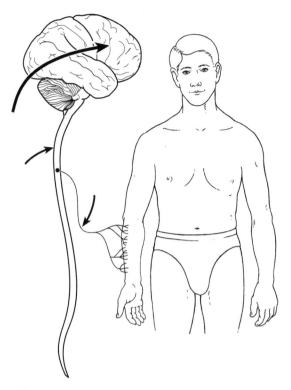

FIGURE 5-3

The ordinary muscles in the body depend on
an electric signal that starts in the brain, and is
transmitted down the spinal cord, and then along
a nerve. If that signal is interrupted at any point
(arrows), the muscle will be paralyzed.

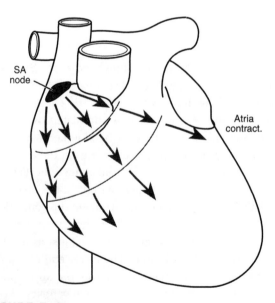

FIGURE 5-4

The heart doesn't depend on the brain to make it beat.
It has its own source of electric energy—the sinoatrial node.
The heartbeat starts when the sinoatrial node fires, sending
a wave of energy across the atria.

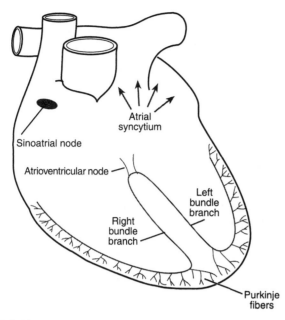

FIGURE 5-5

The conducting tissues of the heart.

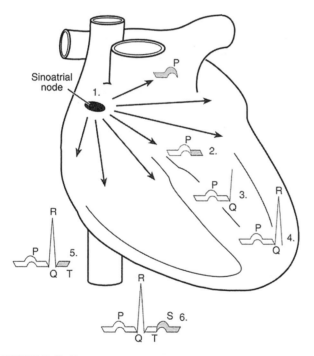

FIGURE 5-6

The waves of the electrocardiogram. **1.** The sinoatrial node discharges, and an activating wave spreads uniformly across the atria. This inscribes the P wave. **2.** The activating wave passes through the AV node, inscribing a flat segment following the P wave. **3.** The activating wave enters the septum, inscribing the first part of the ventricular complex. **4.** The activating wave reaches the extremity of the ventricular network. The remainder of the ventricular complex is inscribed. **5.** A "quiet" period follows ventricular activation, represented by a flat segment. **6.** The wave of repolarization moving back across the heart then inscribes the "recovery" or T wave.

The waves of the electrocardiogram have specific names. Activation of the atria produces the first wave of the heart cycle, a low, rounded wave called a P wave. Then there is a flat segment as the activating impulse moves down the AV node, followed by a series of sharp up-and-down deflections called the Q, R, and S waves. Finally, a restoring current moves through the heart to prepare the cells for the next activation, much like somebody setting up pins in a bowling alley. This restoring or recovery wave is called the T wave, and it ends the electric cycle of the heart (Fig. 5–6).

THE HEART AS AN OXYGEN PUMP

All this marvelous machinery has one function—to deliver oxygen to the tissues. Oxygen is the fuel that drives all animal life. The heart–lung machine pulls oxygen out of the air and into the blood where it is carried to the cells that will use it. It is important to understand exactly how this happens.

The air you breathe is about 20% oxygen; most of the other 80% is nitrogen. Imagine that you could follow a bubble of air down the windpipe (the **trachea**). Soon you would see the single tube divide into two main passages called the **right** and **left bronchi.** These passages again divide into smaller and smaller tubes, exactly like the stems of a bunch of grapes. When the passages become very small they are called **bronchioles,** or "little bronchi." Finally, the bubble ends its course in a tiny spherical sac, like a microscopic grape: this is the air cell or **alveolus,** the almost miraculous structure where oxygen is taken into the blood and waste products leave it (Fig. 5–7).

Imagine that you were about 1/32 of an inch tall, so that you could stand inside the alveolus. You would be looking at a moist, pearl gray wall that you could see through. On the other side of the wall, right against it, you would see a torrent of red fluid rushing past. This is blood (Fig. 5–8).

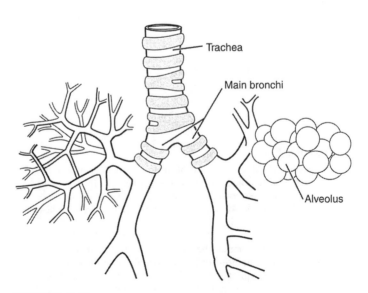

FIGURE 5–7
Basic anatomy of the lung.

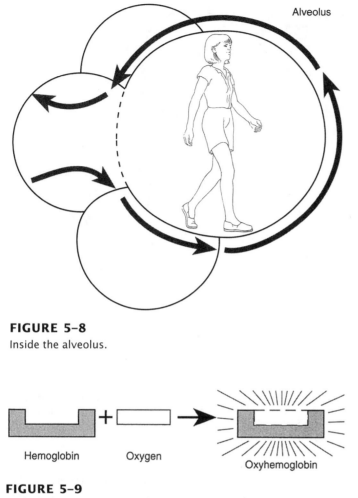

FIGURE 5–8
Inside the alveolus.

Hemoglobin   Oxygen   Oxyhemoglobin

FIGURE 5–9
Oxygenation of hemoglobin.

You would notice that as the blood enters the space around the alveolus it is dark red, but as it leaves it is bright crimson. Oxygen from the alveolus has moved across the thin wall and into the blood, changing its color.

This miraculous exchange is possible because of the pigment in the red blood cells called hemoglobin. It has the ability to pick up oxygen and lock it into its molecules the way a sponge soaks up water. After this happens, the pigment is called oxyhemoglobin (Fig. 5–9).

Oxygen is carried in this form to the cells of the body, where it is released. The oxygen-poor hemoglobin (also called reduced hemoglobin) then returns to the lungs to be recharged.

It's impossible to talk about the delivery of oxygen to the tissues without talking about what comes back from the tissues after the oxygen has been used for fuel. What comes back, of course, is the waste product that's left after the oxygen is burned—carbon dioxide, or CO_2. Carbon dioxide combines with chemicals in the blood to form bicarbonate and carbonic acid. These are two very common chemicals by the way: sodium bicarbonate is the stuff you may have taken for an upset stomach, and carbonic acid is what makes soda water fizz. In these chemical combinations CO_2 is carried to the lungs and released. Carbon dioxide moves easily through the membranes of the blood vessels and the lungs and even with a failing heart, the body can get rid of it (Fig. 5–10).

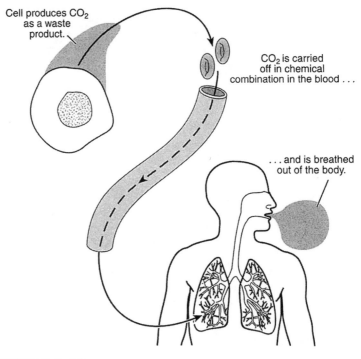

Cell produces CO_2
as a waste
product.

CO_2 is carried
off in chemical
combination in the blood . . .

. . . and is breathed
out of the body.

FIGURE 5–10

Every cell in the body releases carbon dioxide (CO_2) as a waste
product. It is carried away in the blood. The CO_2 reacts to form
two chemicals in the blood—carbonic acid (H_2CO_3) and sodium
bicarbonate ($NaHCO_3$). The chemicals break down in the lungs
to release the CO_2, which is exhaled.

Many forms of disease can interrupt this exchange. The air cells can become scarred
and thickened or can actually rupture as a result of cigarette smoke. (See Chapter 16,
Pulmonary Heart Disease.) Infection can scar the membranes so they can't exchange
oxygen or get rid of CO_2. Failure of the pumping action of the heart can make the lungs so
congested they can't pick up oxygen. Anemia, a condition in which there isn't enough
hemoglobin, can dangerously lower the oxygen-carrying capacity of the blood.

Failure of oxygen delivery and correction of that failure are basic considerations in
almost every kind of heart disease. To understand the heart and heart disease, it is
essential to think of the heart as an oxygen pump.

Heart Failure

Before you consider the failure of a system you have to be sure you know how it works. Try putting together everything you've learned so far.

Imagine you were viewing a functioning model of a human, made of glass so that you could observe everything happening inside. You'd see dark blood rushing through the veins, all over the body, until those veins came together like many streams combining into two rivers—the great superior and inferior cavernous veins (superior and inferior vena cava). You'd see the heart relaxing, pulling that blood into the right ventricle, and then contracting, pumping it out to the lungs. You'd see the blood turn from dark red to bright red in the lungs as it picks up oxygen. Then you'd see the left heart pull this bright red blood out of the lungs and pump it into the body. With each beat, the right heart pumps exactly the same amount of blood **into** the lungs that the left heart pumps **out** (Fig. 6–1).

The valves swing open just in time to permit the rush of blood to the next chamber, or, in other cases, to permit the flow of blood out of the right heart to the lungs and out of the left heart to the body. They snap shut just in time to prevent a backflow or leakage of blood back into the chamber it just left.

You would notice that the motion of blood through the body is very swift: about 6 quarts of blood move completely through the body from the left heart out through the arteries and back to the right heart through the veins in less than a minute. Everything is in a taut, precise balance, synchronized down to a fraction of a drop of blood and a thousandth of a second.

What if something goes wrong?

LEFT HEART FAILURE

To take the simplest example, what if something weakens the left ventricle so that it pumps a little less blood **out** of the lungs with each beat than the right ventricle pumps **in** (Fig. 6–2)? This could happen for many reasons—weakening of the heart muscle, a leaky valve, excessively high blood pressure. Imagine that the difference is as little as a drop and try some simple arithmetic to see what happens.

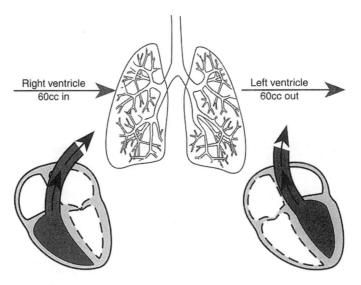

FIGURE 6-1
Normally the right ventricle pumps the same amount of blood into
the lungs with each beat that the left ventricle pumps out.

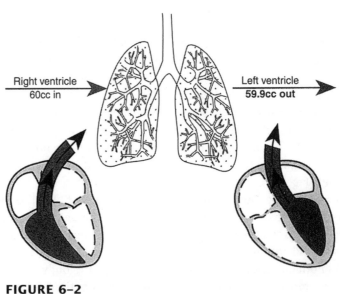

FIGURE 6-2
Left heart failure. If the left ventricle falls behind by as little as
one drop with each beat, a large amount of blood can "pile up" in
the lungs in a few hours.

A drop of blood equals about 0.1 cubic centimeter (cc). If the heart is beating 80 times a minute, there will be 8 cc of extra blood trapped in the lungs in 1 minute. In 1 hour there will be almost a pint of extra blood trapped in the lungs. This extra volume of blood will compress the small air passages. In addition, watery fluid will leak out of the overloaded capillaries into the tissue spaces between the air passages, with further compression.

There won't be room for a normal exchange of air, and the patient will become short of breath (Fig. 6–3). (The medical term for shortness of breath—**dyspnea**—comes

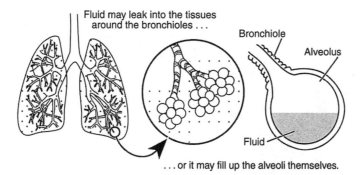

Fluid may leak into the tissues
around the bronchioles . . .

Bronchiole

Alveolus

Fluid

. . . or it may fill up the alveoli themselves.

FIGURE 6–3
This extra pressure of blood in the small vessels of the lungs
forces watery fluid out of the blood vessels and into the tissues of
the lungs. Fluid may distend the tissues around the air passages,
or it may enter the alveoli.

from the Greek stem *dys*, implying "abnormal" or "difficult," and *pneumon*, meaning
"air.") **Thus there is only one symptom of failure of the left ventricle: shortness of
breath, or dyspnea**.

This dyspnea can take several forms. It may appear very gradually, so that a golfer
notes that he has to stop more often to get his breath, until one day he can hardly walk
to the first tee. The patient, in effect, has become seriously disabled. This process can
take weeks or it may progress very rapidly, in a matter of days, to the point at which
the patient is confined to a chair or to a bed.

The dyspnea of left heart failure can take a terrifying, life-threatening form. The
process of engorgement of the lungs can progress so rapidly that the air cells or alveoli
actually fill with fluid. This condition is called **acute pulmonary edema** and it is a gen-
uine medical emergency. The victim often wakens at night gasping, blue, and near
death: the fluid has been quietly accumulating during sleep, and by the time the patient
wakens there is barely enough oxygen exchange to sustain life. Without medical treatment, acute pulmonary edema is always fatal; with adequate medical measures, the
patient can be out of danger in 10 or 15 minutes. ("Adequate medical measures" include
one step that can be carried on by anyone, in any setting. See Chapters 19 and 22.)

RIGHT HEART FAILURE

Sometimes the right heart can't pump the blood out to the lungs as fast as it rushes in
from the veins. This could happen because the valve leading out of the right heart to
the lungs was diseased, scarred, or partly closed. Most commonly it happens because
of chronic disease in the lungs, so that the resistance in the blood vessels of the lungs
is abnormally high (Fig. 6–4).

Regardless of the cause, the right heart fails, and the blood backs up into the veins
of the body. When the pressure in the veins is abnormally high, water is forced out of
the veins and into the surrounding tissues: it's important to note that this fluid accumulates in the spaces between the cells of the body, not inside the cells themselves.
The swelling that results is called **edema**. Since water runs downhill, even inside the
body, the fluid will accumulate in the lowest part of the body—usually the feet. As the
condition grows more severe, the swelling may move upward, with massive accumula-
tion of fluid in the abdomen. Because the fluid of cardiac edema always accumulates in

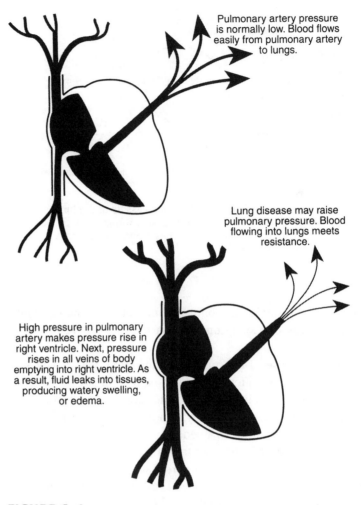

Pulmonary artery pressure is normally low. Blood flows easily from pulmonary artery to lungs.

Lung disease may raise pulmonary pressure. Blood flowing into lungs meets resistance.

High pressure in pulmonary artery makes pressure rise in right ventricle. Next, pressure rises in all veins of body emptying into right ventricle. As a result, fluid leaks into tissues, producing watery swelling, or edema.

FIGURE 6–4
Pulmonary edema.

the lowest part of the body, it is called **dependent edema. Thus there is only one finding in right heart failure: dependent edema.**

The terms **left heart failure, right heart failure, congestive failure, dyspnea,** and **edema** will be used frequently throughout the rest of the book. Be sure you're comfortable with them before leaving this chapter.

CHAPTER 7

Hypertensive Heart Disease

DEFINITION OF HYPERTENSION

The word **hypertension** means "high blood pressure." (It has nothing to do with being nervous or agitated.)

Liquid always exerts pressure on the walls of whatever is holding it. When you fill a glass with water, the water presses against the sides of the glass with a certain measurable force (Fig. 7–1A).

In the same way, the blood presses against the walls of the blood vessels with a definite, measurable force called the blood pressure. The term **blood pressure** refers to the pressure in the arteries, not the veins (Fig. 7–1B).

The pressure in the arteries rises and falls with each heartbeat. It rises when the heart contracts, pumping blood into the arteries. It falls during diastole, when no blood is being pumped out of the heart. This change in pressure is what makes it possible to feel a pulse (Fig. 7–2).

With the sphygmomanometer, or blood pressure cuff, it is possible to measure the peak of systolic pressure and the bottom of diastolic pressure. The cuff is inflated with air until it is well over the systolic pressure and then is slowly deflated. When the pressure in the cuff equals the peak pressure in the arteries, a snapping sound will be heard as the blood forces the vessel open at peak pressure only to have it collapse between beats. The sound is produced when the walls of the artery snap shut. All sound will disappear when the pressure in the cuff equals the lowest pressure since the vessel will then stay open throughout the heart cycle. The pressure is described as systolic over diastolic—for example, 120/80.

Question: 120 what? *Answer:* 120 millimeters of mercury (mm Hg). Blood pressure is measured by the height of a column of mercury in a glass tube that the blood pressure will support.

"Normal" blood pressure? You might as well ask "what is a normal height?" There's a wide range of normal, and everyone's blood pressure changes from minute to minute. It will rise with excitement or exercise; it may fall during sleep or rest or even on standing from a sitting position. For an average adult, a systolic pressure between 100 and 140 is normal. Diastolic pressure will lie between 60 and 90. A thin, young female or a

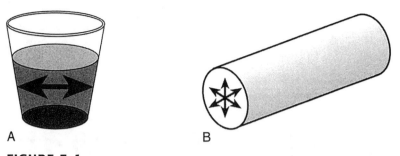

FIGURE 7-1

A. Pressure exerted on walls of container. **B.** Blood pressing against walls of vessel.

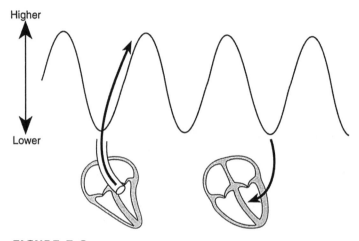

FIGURE 7-2

Blood pressure goes up and down in accord with the cardiac cycle of systole and diastole.

highly trained athlete might have a systolic pressure under 90 with no ill effects while a healthy 60-year-old might have a pressure of 156/90 as a normal finding (Fig. 7–3).

KINDS OF HYPERTENSION

The arteries aren't just passive tubes. They are living organs with nerves and strong muscles: they can expand or constrict with the speed and power of a snake. Normal arteries are elastic; they have a lot of "give." By expanding when blood is pumped out of the heart and contracting during diastole, they help to equalize pressure during the heart cycle.

In older patients, the arteries may become rigid and pipelike. Now the vessels are like a boxer who can't "roll with the punches." With no give in the system, the systolic pressure will be abnormally high. The diastolic pressure will remain normal. This is **systolic hypertension**; it was formerly thought to be harmless, but we now know that it isn't (Fig. 7–4A).

If the arteries become constricted and stay that way, the blood pumped out of the heart is forced into a smaller container. The pressure has to rise. Both systolic and diastolic pressures go up. This is **diastolic hypertension**—it may be dangerous and it always needs treatment (Fig. 7–4B).

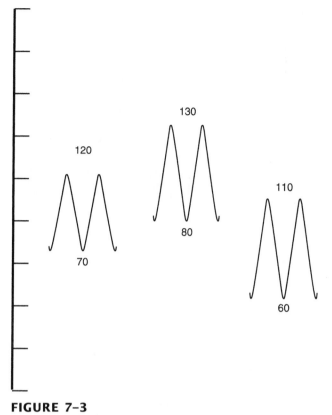

FIGURE 7–3

The range of normal blood pressure. Blood pressure changes from hour to hour and from person to person. One cannot say that a given figure is exactly "normal." The physician must evaluate the pressure in relation to the patient's age, weight, and medical condition.

COMPLICATIONS OF HYPERTENSION

Hypertension is a dangerous disease because it can produce three major, potentially lethal complications.

Congestive Heart Failure

Imagine a worker who has the job of pumping water up a 20-foot (ft) pipe. He can do this easily. Suddenly he's asked to pump water up a 10-story building. The effort of pumping against the enormous increase in pressure will wear him out. For a time his muscles will enlarge as he struggles with the abnormal load, but finally, he'll be exhausted and he won't be able to pump water out of his pipe as fast as it flows in. The water will back up and there will be flooding somewhere in the system. This is exactly what happens to the left ventricle when it has to pump against a high pressure. At first the muscle wall thickens in an attempt to compensate (Fig. 7–5), but finally the heart fails: it can't pump blood out into the aorta as fast as it runs in from the lungs, and the pressure backs up into the lungs with congestive heart failure. This can happen abruptly: it is common to see a hypertensive patient who has been substantially free of symptoms suddenly go into massive pulmonary edema. Most cardiologists would probably tell you this is statistically the commonest cause of abrupt, life-threatening left heart failure. It is not clear why the break in cardiac compensation is so abrupt or

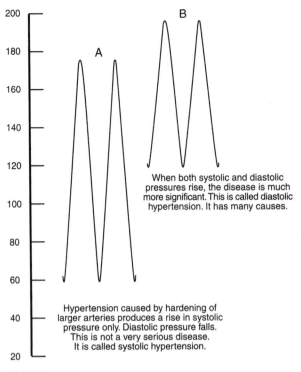

When both systolic and diastolic pressures rise, the disease is much more significant. This is called diastolic hypertension. It has many causes.

Hypertension caused by hardening of larger arteries produces a rise in systolic pressure only. Diastolic pressure falls. This is not a very serious disease. It is called systolic hypertension.

FIGURE 7–4

Hypertension caused by hardening of the larger arteries produces a rise in systolic pressure only. Diastolic pressure is unchanged or may actually fall. This condition, called systolic hypertension, was formerly considered a benign entity, but we now know it can cause problems if untreated.

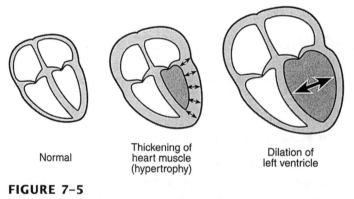

Normal

Thickening of heart muscle (hypertrophy)

Dilation of left ventricle

FIGURE 7–5

Left ventricle response in severe hypertension.

why patients tolerate a high blood pressure so long without warning symptoms, but the phenomenon of sudden, life-threatening pulmonary edema in a hypertensive patient is familiar to every emergency department physician.

Stroke

The word **stroke** is the same as the medical term **cerebrovascular accident**. It means that the blood supply to some part of the brain has been cut off. This can happen because a blood vessel ruptures and bleeds or because a vessel becomes plugged in some way. Hypertension puts an enormous strain on the smaller arteries, and they can simply rupture. The result is like having a nosebleed in the brain: a certain amount of brain tissue loses its blood supply and the cells die. When the blood supply to brain cells is cut off, they begin to die within 10 minutes. The effect on the patient, of course, depends on which cells are affected: there may be paralysis of major parts of the body or there may be no more than a temporary blurring of consciousness.

It's frightening to think that the effects of a stroke are a matter of simple chance—the results depend on which blood vessel ruptures and where in its course the rupture occurs. Hypertension was once the commonest cause of stroke, but with better medical agents and better treatment there has been a very encouraging drop in the occurrence of hypertensive strokes in recent years. In fact, the partial conquest of hypertensive stroke has been one of the major advances of modern medicine, much more important in long-term effect than all the spectacular advances in cardiac surgery.

Coronary Artery Disease

The cells that form the lining of the coronary arteries are often damaged when the pressure within the vessel is abnormally high. They begin to degenerate, and masses of fat, or **atheromas**, are likely to form, tending to block the flow of blood through the vessel (Fig. 7–6). Patients with hypertension face at least a 200% increase in risk of coronary artery disease. Why does hypertension affect the lining of the coronary arteries? The answer is not at all clear, but the association is established beyond question. Does control of blood pressure prevent coronary disease? It's reasonable to think so, but the results so far are not as clear-cut as in the prevention of stroke: more data are needed.

Kidney Failure

This is a "chicken-and-egg" situation. High blood pressure can certainly produce damage in the blood vessels of the kidneys, often with severe kidney failure. On the other hand, kidney disease can produce high blood pressure. Sometimes it is hard to tell which caused which.

When an intelligent physician detects high blood pressure, it's not an end point; it's the signal for a swift clinical investigation:

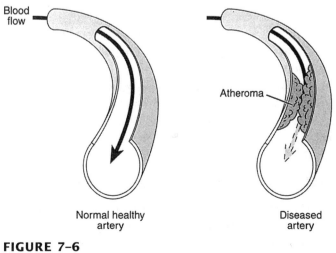

Blood flow

Atheroma

Normal healthy artery

Diseased artery

FIGURE 7–6
Fatty plaque blocking a coronary artery.

What kind of hypertension is present? Mild and relatively benign? Severe and
    dangerous?

What associated diseases are present?

What complications are present?

Can a specific cause be found?

    Note: *Practically all these complications can be prevented by controlling high blood
pressure.*

VARIETIES OF HYPERTENSION: CAUSES AND TREATMENT

Modern understanding of hypertension began when a physician named Goldblatt put a
clamp on the renal artery of a dog, cutting down the blood flow to the kidney. When he
did, the dog's blood pressure went up. Extensive research showed that when the kidney tissue wasn't receiving an adequate blood supply, a chemical called renin was
released into the bloodstream in large amounts. This chemical acts as an enzyme split-
ting certain proteins to produce a substance called angiotensin I. Still another enzyme
converts this substance to angiotensin II, a powerful agent that causes constriction of
the small arteries and a rise in blood pressure. While this reaction was first detected
when a kidney was deliberately damaged, years of study have shown that this inter-
play of chemicals is the basis of a great deal of hypertension even when there is no kidney disease. This isn't the only mechanism of hypertension, but it's a very important
one and will reappear throughout this chapter. Some studies have concentrated on the
effect of chemicals released at nerve endings in the walls of small blood vessels,
whereas others have correlated changes in the anatomy of arteries with hypertension.
All these elements play a role in treatment and outcome.

    The great majority of patients with severe kidney disease will suffer from hyper-
tension, but the reverse is not true. Only a small minority of cases of hypertension are
caused by kidney disease.

ESSENTIAL HYPERTENSION

In about 90% of cases, there's no cause for hypertension anyone can find. The medical
profession calls these cases "essential hypertension." (Beautiful word, *essential*—it's
mysterious, impressive, and totally insignificant. If a patient had a high fever for no
known reason, the diagnosis of essential hyperpyrexia would probably make everyone
feel a lot better, but all it really says is that the patient has a fever and the physician
doesn't know why.) In a small minority of cases, a specific cause of hypertension can
be detected: kidney disease, tumors of the adrenal gland, or congenital abnormalities;
these will be described later. At this point, it's important to concentrate on the vast
majority of cases in the essential group.

Salt and Essential Hypertension

A few years ago anthropologists discovered a tribe in the Amazon jungles that never
used salt because it was taboo. The minerals in the blood of these Indians showed an
unusual pattern: the potassium level was unusually high and the sodium level was very
low. Nobody in the tribe had high blood pressure. Salt isn't the whole story, but there

is no question that too much salt tends to raise blood pressure and severe salt restriction lowers it. Before modern drugs were available, many cases of hypertension were controlled simply by cutting the salt in the diet to a very low level (200 milligrams [mg] of sodium). This isn't a diet anyone would choose to eat (it's mostly rice) and such a diet isn't needed anymore, but it does illustrate the importance of salt in hypertension.

Avoidance of excess amounts of sodium is a simple, obvious first step in treatment of hypertension. Salt substitutes are available to season food. In addition, the hypertensive patient should avoid "junk food," which is loaded with sodium, and obvious sources of salt like ham or bacon. Over-the-counter home remedies like antacids also should be checked for sodium content.

Diuretic drugs, or drugs that cause salt and water to move out of the body, have been an important part of the treatment of hypertension since the sixties. For years they were considered "first-line" drugs; they certainly are effective in lowering blood pressure in many patients. However, there are undesirable side effects. They drain essential minerals like potassium and magnesium and they often have a bad effect on blood fats and blood sugar. As a result the diuretic agents are being replaced by newer, more powerful drugs with fewer side effects.

Changes in the Arteries

Generally speaking, there are two kinds of change in the arteries that may raise blood pressure. The first is the general "hardening" that often goes with age. The walls of the arteries are infiltrated with rigid elements so that the vessels resemble tire casing instead of flexible rubber (Fig. 7–7). There are whole volumes of theories about why this happens, but nobody really knows the answer. This results in systolic hypertension.

Second, and much more serious, is the "scared snake" phenomenon: arteries that are structurally normal suddenly become oversensitive to certain elements that circulate in the body: they constrict powerfully and they stay constricted. Of course, the blood pressure rises. It's important to know what these elements are because blocking their effect is the key to treatment of high blood pressure.

Adrenaline and Other Catecholamines

Consider a remote ancestor—back about the year 1,000,000 B.C. Gramps came face-to-face with a cave bear and it was clear that one of them was not going to walk away. As he swung his club and reached for a rock, certain changes took place that made him ready for fight or flight. His adrenal glands pumped a lot of adrenaline and other chemicals like adrenaline into his blood: the same chemicals were released from nerve endings all over his body. These chemicals—adrenaline and its cousins—are called **catecholamines**. Note this name well.

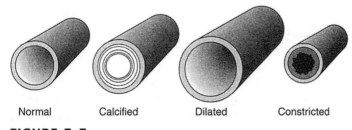

Normal   Calcified   Dilated   Constricted

FIGURE 7–7
Harmful arterial changes.

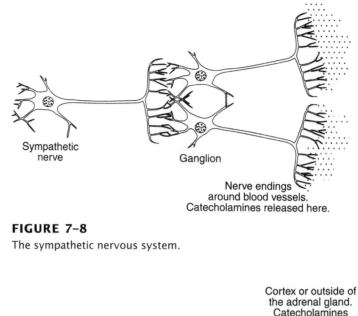

FIGURE 7–8
The sympathetic nervous system.

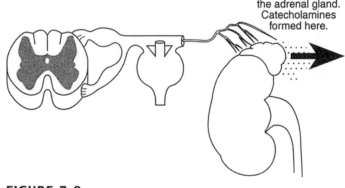

FIGURE 7–9
The adrenal glands, situated above the kidneys, also produce catecholamines. They are released directly into blood and circulate to stimulate the receptors in the various organs.

The catecholamines made his arteries constrict so that his blood pressure rose: his heart beat faster and pumped more blood. His muscles were supercharged and he may have involuntarily emptied his bowels or his bladder. In every way he was prepared for the fight. In your ancestor's case, it worked, because here you are. He either killed the bear or got up a tree: either way, the catecholamine surge helped him.

Catecholamines are formed in two places—at the endings of the sympathetic nerves (Fig. 7–8) and in the adrenal glands, the small glands that lie right above the kidneys (Fig. 7–9). A number of drugs are now available to block the effects of catecholamines. They act at different places along the delivery chain.

Catecholamine-Blocking Drugs: How and Where They Act

Methyldopa and clonidine act in the central nervous system. Certain types of activity in the brain actually send out messages that cause an increase in the intensity of the impulses traveling down the nerves to increase the release of catecholamines at the nerve endings. Methyldopa and clonidine actually block or reduce the stimulation before it can travel down the nerves. Two other substances, reserpine and guanethidine,

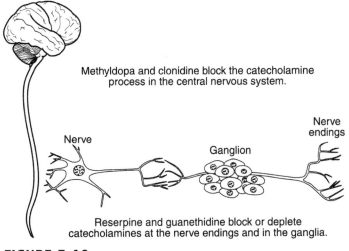

Methyldopa and clonidine block the catecholamine process in the central nervous system.

Nerve endings

Nerve

Ganglion

Nerve endings

Reserpine and guanethidine block or deplete catecholamines at the nerve endings and in the ganglia.

FIGURE 7–10
Sites of action of catecholamine blockers.

block release of catecholamines at the other end of the chain—at the nerve endings themselves (Fig. 7–10).

When catecholamines are released at the nerve endings they act on the cells in the arterial wall. These cells have certain **receiving elements**, or **receptors**, that enable the cells to react to the catecholamines. There are two types of receptor elements at the end of the sympathetic nerve chain. They are called alpha (α) receptors and beta (β) receptors, and they have very different effects when stimulated. Drugs that block the beta receptors cause the blood pressure to fall for reasons that are not entirely clear. Beta-blocking drugs (propranolol, metoprolol, atenolol, and others) are very useful in treating hypertension and other kinds of heart disease. Alpha-receptor blockers like prazosin cause direct dilatation of both arteries and veins. These agents are excellent antihypertensive drugs with few if any significant side effects. Prazosin blocks the alpha receptors and thus causes direct dilatation of both arteries and veins.

ACE Inhibitors

Earlier in the chapter you read about the role of renin in the production of hypertension. Renin acts indirectly by helping to break down a circulating protein called angiotensinogen. The result of this reaction is angiotensin I. This substance is then broken down in the lungs with the help of a catalyzing enzyme called angiotensin-converting enzyme (ACE); the final result is angiotensin II, an active chemical that causes constriction of small arteries (Fig. 7–11). Drugs known as ACE inhibitors are able to lower the blood pressure by blocking formation of ACE in the lungs, thereby reducing the level of angiotensin II in the bloodstream. They are effective in about 50% of cases.

Direct Dilators

A number of drugs act directly on the cells in the arterial wall to make them relax so that the vessel dilates and the blood pressure falls. Whether the constriction is caused by catecholamines or angiotensin II, the direct dilators will dilate the arteries because they act directly on the muscle cells in the walls of the vessels (Fig. 7–12). Drugs in this class include minoxidil, nitroprusside, and hydralazine.

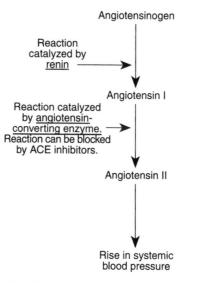

FIGURE 7-11
How renin affects the production of angiotensin II.

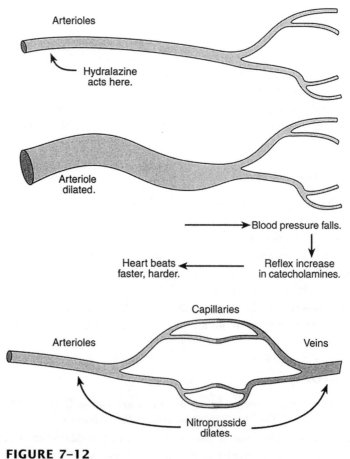

FIGURE 7-12
Direct vasodilators.

Calcium Blockers

The calcium ion has powerful metabolic effects throughout the body. In the heart, it is directly involved in the chemistry of muscle contraction; movement of calcium ions into the fibers of the heart muscle is a key element in the chain that leads to normal contraction. In general, calcium ions have a tendency to produce contraction of heart muscle cells and constriction of blood vessel walls. **Calcium-blocking agents**, therefore, can be expected to cause relaxation and dilatation of the arterioles, and this is exactly what they do. Calcium-blocking agents are very useful in the treatment of hypertension and by now the drug companies have produced a whole spectrum of them.

Spironolactone

One of the pleasant surprises of the past few years has been the effectiveness of this chemical in controlling hypertension. Spironolactone was thought of as a diuretic, which it is, but by blocking the effect of aldosterone, an adrenal secretion, spironolactone has emerged as a dramatically effective agent in controlling hypertension—even in difficult and refractory cases.

Combined Therapy

It is often necessary to use combinations of drugs to control hypertension or to balance the effects of the various agents. Some of the dilators, like hydralazine, can make the heart beat too rapidly: a beta-blocking drug is useful at that point to slow it. Both drugs, of course, tend to decrease blood pressure so that the combined effect can be very beneficial. Table 17–1 lists the leading antihypertensive drugs and tells how and where they act. Like all potent agents, the antihypertensive drugs often have undesirable side effects; these are listed in Table 17–2.

Weight Loss

Obesity causes hypertension. Losing weight lowers elevated blood pressure. If an overweight hypertensive person loses as little as 10 or 15 pounds the pressure will often drop abruptly. Nobody is quite sure why this happens, but there is no question that it does. There's an ironic twist here, however; few fat people lose weight permanently. In some of the best controlled studies at major medical centers, only 10% of obese people lost weight and kept it off.

The current obsession with health and weight control may change this picture. Any fat hypertensive person should be directed to an organized, supervised weight control program and it should be pushed with fanatical zeal. Casual advice to "cut back on the calories" is a waste of everyone's time. The health care worker who does not move heaven and earth to make fat hypertensive people lose weight has shirked a critical obligation.

Two Dangerous Variations of the Disease

Accelerated or Malignant Hypertension

A patient between 30 and 60 years of age presents with headaches, blurred vision, shortness of breath, or chest pain. The diastolic pressure is over 110. The blood vessels of both retinas show severe disease with hemorrhages, spots of dead material that look like cotton wool, and bulging of the optic nerve into the eye (papilledema). This is

TABLE 7-1   Summary of Antihypertensive Drugs: Where They Act and How

Classes of agents	Effects
Diuretics	
Thiazides (chlorthiazide and related drugs) Thiazidelike sulfonilamide compounds (chlorthalidone, metolazone, etc.) Loop diuretics (bumetanide, ethacrynic acid) Furosemide	All these drugs cause the kidneys to excrete large quantities of sodium and water. Furosemide is very potent, but is too short-acting for routine hypertensive treatment.
Potassium-sparing agents (spironolactone and related drugs)	These drugs are weaker diuretics, but they prevent the excessive loss of potassium that takes place with other diuretics.
Catecholamine-blocking drugs	
Methyldopa, clonidine, and guanabenz (central blockers) Reserpine, guanethidine (peripheral blockers) Phenoxybenzamine, phentolamine (α-receptor blockers) Propranolol, atenolol, metoprolol, timolol (β-receptor blockers)	All these drugs block the effects of catecholamines on the small arteries. The α- and β-blockers block certain specific undesirable side effects.
ACE inhibitors	
Captopril, enalapril, lisinopril	These drugs block the formation of angiotensin II from renin. The effect is to relax the smaller arteries and lower pressure.
Calcium blockers	
Verapamil, nifedipine, diltiazem, nicardipine	By blocking movement of calcium ions, these drugs dilate the smaller arteries and lower pressure.
Direct dilators	
Hydralazine, minoxidil, nitroprusside	Direct action on smooth muscle of smallest arteries (precapillaries). Untoward effects of hydralazine and minoxidil must often be balanced with diuretics and beta blockers. Nitroprusside (IV only) dilates both arteries and veins.

the picture of accelerated or malignant hypertension. There is a 50% chance of severe associated kidney disease. Patients with these findings should always be hospitalized and treated vigorously. Even with the best treatment, 30% will die in 1 to 2 years, and 50% will die in 5 years. Anyone involved in the care of hypertensive patients must be aware of this dangerous subtype of the disease: it's easy to recognize and it constitutes a real emergency.

Hypertensive Crisis

Every health care worker should know what a hypertensive crisis is; so should every patient who suffers from hypertension. It's another life-and-death emergency and it's remarkably easy to recognize.

First, there's a sudden rise in blood pressure with a high diastolic pressure (240/120, for example). Second, there's evidence that the high blood pressure is affecting the brain or the heart. The effect on the brain can be severe—a massive stroke with loss of consciousness, for example—or it may be so mild that the patient is only aware of severe dizziness, difficulty speaking, or weakness of some muscles. The important point is that there are suddenly symptoms of some kind of impaired brain function. If

TABLE 7-2 Undesirable Side Effects of Some Commonly Used Antihypertensive Drugs	
Classes of agents	**Effects**
Catecholamine-blocking drugs	
Reserpine	Nasal congestion, drowsiness, gastric ulceration (rare), nightmares
Alpha-methyldopa (Aldomet)	Sedation, dry mouth, hypotension, impotence
Clonidine (Catapres)	Sedation, dry mouth, dangerous tendency to "overshoot" with rise in pressure when drug is abruptly discontinued
Prazosin (Minipress)	Excessive drop in pressure with first dose; few other toxic effects
Beta-blocking drugs	Depression of ventricular function, depression of sinus node function and AV nodal conduction; worsening of asthma, COPD, peripheral vascular disease, diabetes
Diuretic agents	
Hydrochlorothiazide, furosemide, ethacrynic acid	Loss of potassium, magnesium; elevation of blood sugar, lipids, and uric acid
Spironolactone	Originally used as a diuretic, now a major antihypertensive; problem is potassium *retention*
Vasodilators	
Hydralazine	Tachycardia, flushing, headache, precipitation of angina (all controllable with concomitant use of beta blockers)
Minoxidil	As above, plus a tendency to excessive hair growth
Calcium blockers	
Verapamil	Serious depression of left ventricular function; AV block
Diltiazem	Minimal effect on AV nodal conduction and left ventricular function
Nifedipine, nicardipine	Same
ACE inhibitors	
Captopril, enalapril, lisinopril	Severe, intractable cough in about 10%–15% of patients; worsening of some types of kidney disease; angioneurotic edema

the heart is affected, the patient will describe one of two symptoms—chest pain (angina) or shortness of breath (congestive heart failure)—or, sometimes, both.

Treatment. "Hypertensive emergency" is a good title for these two conditions. The first part of treatment is a swift trip to the nearest hospital. This is not a condition that can be treated at home. Second, the blood pressure is lowered gradually, in controlled steps. Nitroprusside, given by vein, is the ideal drug for this purpose. It can be controlled precisely and there is no real danger of overreaction: the drug is gone within 2 or 3 minutes after the infusion is stopped. The blood pressure is lowered in carefully controlled steps of 10 to 20 mm every few minutes. The physician must, however, observe for worsening of symptoms at each level.

Worsening? Why should the patient get worse when the blood pressure falls? Consider plumbing. The amount of fluid flowing through a pipe depends on two things: the size of the pipe and the pressure driving the fluid.

If the pipe is narrowed, like a hardened artery, it takes more pressure to push the same amount of fluid through it. When the pressure has been high for some time, the

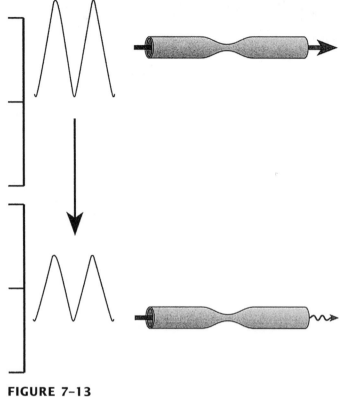

FIGURE 7-13
Abrupt fall in pressure.

blood vessels and tissues will be "set" for this kind of pressure to maintain flow. You might say that parts of the body have become "used to" a high-driving pressure in the arteries. When the pressure falls too abruptly, the amount of blood reaching certain parts of the brain or the heart may fall below the critical level. The patient may suffer a stroke or a heart attack (Fig. 7–13).

Certain drugs will drop blood pressure very quickly: diazoxide can be given by vein, or a calcium-blocking drug called nifedipine may be given in a quickly absorbed tablet under the tongue. These drugs should NEVER be used in a hypertensive crisis. Once they are in the body, their effect cannot be "turned off" or neutralized and the patient may easily suffer a stroke or heart attack or die with little hope of remedy.

Nitroprusside, on the other hand, can be controlled as precisely as a setscrew, and its effect can be reversed in a few seconds. It is the ideal drug to control a hypertensive crisis.

Rare Types of Hypertension

Renal or Kidney Hypertension

If kidney tissue doesn't get enough blood, a large amount of renin is released into the circulation. Renin, of course, breaks down into angiotensins and blood pressure rises. Hardening of the renal artery leading into a kidney can do this; so can certain types of kidney disease that produce scarring and constriction of kidney tissue. An abrupt rise in pressure in someone age 50 or older should always raise suspicion of kidney disease as the cause. Hardening in a renal artery can now be corrected with a catheter, without

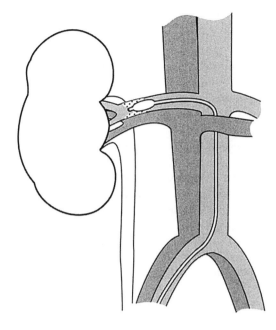

FIGURE 7–14
Use of a balloon catheter to clear an obstruction
in a renal artery.

surgery, so the possibility of curing some of these cases is very reasonable (Fig. 7–14). Possibly 2% of all cases of hypertension are specifically caused by kidney disease.

Adrenal Hypertension

The adrenal glands make catecholamines and cortisols (cortisone and related chemicals). Either of these normal hormone groups, in excess, can cause hypertension. Pheochromocytoma is the impressive name of a benign tumor of the catecholamine-forming cells of the adrenal gland. Catecholamines are released in surges, the blood pressure soars to dangerous heights, and the patient is usually aware of symptoms like headache, dizziness, or chest pain. It's not too difficult to diagnose this condition since there are specific tests for levels of catecholamines in the blood and urine. Pheochromocytoma should be suspected whenever patients suffer from sudden paroxysms of severe hypertension. After proper medical treatment these tumors can be removed easily and safely, with complete cure of the hypertension.

Adrenocortical Adenoma

Other types of benign (noncancerous) growths in the outside, or cortex, of the adrenal gland can cause high blood pressure. These tumors manufacture a type of cortisone that causes the body to retain abnormal amounts of salt and water, and hypertension follows. Again, this rare form of hypertension can be cured by surgery.

Final Note: *The conquest of hypertension is one of the great medical achievements of the 20th century. Now that almost all cases of hypertension can be controlled, the physician faces a challenge of awesome proportions. Anyone caring for hypertensive patients must be prepared to use informed judgment in selecting agents for treatment; to observe carefully for side effects; and to provide a program of prolonged, organized supervision to make sure that the blood pressure goes to normal and stays there.*

Prevention of disease is a thousand times more important than "patching up" after a disaster, and control of elevated blood pressure is prevention par excellence. The effect of this kind of control on death and disease is only now becoming apparent but it is safe to say that the control of elevated blood pressure has provided more net benefit to humanity than the combined efforts of all the cardiac surgeons in medical history. If this chapter helps hypertensive patients or those who care for them attain the goals of normal blood pressure it will be the most important section in the book.

Notes for Critical Care Personnel

Note especially the warnings about dropping seriously elevated blood pressure too fast. It's surprising how many of the new medical generation don't realize the dangers involved. Every standard textbook of medicine and cardiology carries the same warning. Without exception, every authority in the field makes the following recommendations:

1. In the presence of accelerated hypertension or hypertensive crisis,
2. Or when severe hypertension is present in a patient with known or suspected coronary or cerebral vascular disease,
3. Or in older patients when some cardiac or cerebral vascular disease is likely, **lower blood pressure in gradual steps of 15 to 20 mm Hg. Watch the patient for evidence of cerebral or myocardial hypoperfusion at each step (e.g., watch for angina or neurologic changes).**

A few years ago intravenous diazoxide was popular; it dropped blood pressure precipitously and everybody learned the old lesson all over again. After enough patients suffered strokes and myocardial infarcts it fell out of favor. Sublingual nifedipine was used for a time in the same setting but it has been discontinued because it too can cause a swift fall in blood pressure that can result in a stroke or a heart attack. This drug also drops blood pressure in a swift, uncontrolled fashion with the same dangers and complications.

When a patient presents with a combination of crescendo angina or myocardial infarction and severe hypertension, it's critical to lower the blood pressure and it's equally critical to do it carefully and under control. Nitroprusside is the ideal drug here, as it is in most acute hypertensive situations.

Intravenous nitroglycerin is often used but its effect on arterial pressure is variable and often weak. Nitroprusside is powerful, predictable, and easily controllable. (It has a half-life of a few minutes.)

Don't forget that blood pressure is a dynamic, changing phenomenon. One measurement in the supine position may be misleading. Check pressure in various positions and after light activity, such as walking around the room, if possible. The results are often surprising and very informative.

When a patient taking an ACE inhibitor complains of a severe cough it's probably not the flu. These superb agents have one serious drawback—in 10% to 20% of patients they irritate the bronchial surfaces and produce a distressing cough.

CHAPTER 8

Coronary Artery Disease

This chapter will answer five questions:

1. What is coronary artery disease and what actually happens in a diseased coronary artery?
2. What effect does this disease have on the heart and on the body as a whole?
3. How can coronary artery disease be diagnosed?
4. How is coronary artery disease treated?
5. What causes coronary artery disease and how can it be prevented?

Be sure to review the anatomy and names of the major branches of coronary arteries and the abbreviations used to describe them in Chapter 4 (LMCA: left main coronary artery; LAD: left anterior descending branch of the left main vessel; LCA: left circumflex branch of the main left vessel; RCA: right coronary artery).

Now study Figures 8–1 and 8–2. You are looking at illustrations of the major cause of death and invalidism in the Western world. These hard masses of fat obstruct the flow of blood through the coronary arteries. Sometimes the blood flow is cut down so much that the heart muscle is injured; sometimes the vessel is completely blocked and the heart muscle dies. The various clinical forms of coronary artery disease are all the result of this basic process.

TYPES OF DISEASE PRODUCED BY CORONARY ATHEROMATOSIS

Angina Pectoris

Effort Angina

Atheromas (fat deposits within the walls of arteries) form silently. The patient has no way of knowing they exist until they're large enough to form a significant obstruction to the flow of blood through one or more coronary arteries. What does "significant" mean (Fig. 8–3)?

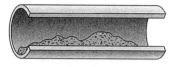
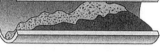

An atheroma is a mass of fat
that forms on the wall of an artery,
partly blocking the vessel.

End view of a partially plugged
coronary artery. Blood flow
through this artery would be
cut down about 50%.

FIGURE 8–1
Coronary atheroma.

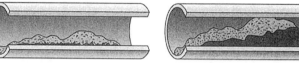

The tissue in the wall
of the coronary artery
under the atheroma may
bleed, or hemorrhage.

The blood may "cut under"
the atheroma and lift
it out into the artery,
blocking it completely.

An abscess or localized
infection may form in the
wall of the coronary artery
under the atheroma.

A blood clot, or thrombus,
often forms over or around
an atheroma. The term
coronary thrombosis means
that the coronary artery
is blocked by a blood clot.

FIGURE 8–2
Complications of coronary atheroma.

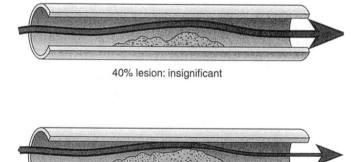

40% lesion: insignificant

70% lesion: danger!

FIGURE 8–3
Atheromas.

Seventy percent is the magic number. When the atheroma grows to about 70% of the diameter of a coronary artery, it may begin to produce symptoms. The reason is that at this point the blood flow to some area of heart muscle will be barely enough for the needs of that muscle when the patient is at rest and the heart isn't working very

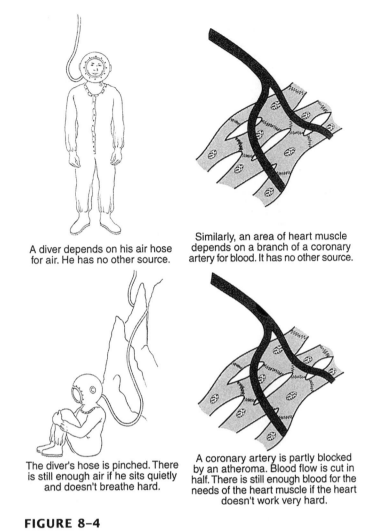

A diver depends on his air hose for air. He has no other source.

Similarly, an area of heart muscle depends on a branch of a coronary artery for blood. It has no other source.

The diver's hose is pinched. There is still enough air if he sits quietly and doesn't breathe hard.

A coronary artery is partly blocked by an atheroma. Blood flow is cut in half. There is still enough blood for the needs of the heart muscle if the heart doesn't work very hard.

FIGURE 8–4
Coronary artery disease and the heart muscle.

hard. When the heart has to beat faster or when it has to work against a higher pressure, it needs more fuel—blood. It can't get the extra fuel it needs because of the narrowing in the coronary artery, and the syndrome called **angina pectoris** results. Study the diver in Figures 8–4, 8–5, and 8–6. Note that in Figure 8–5A he's tugging on the hose pipe to let someone know he's not getting enough air. Heart muscle that's not getting enough blood will often send a message by means of a symptom. The symptom of angina pectoris is painful discomfort somewhere in the upper half of the body: the discomfort comes on with exertion and is relieved by rest.

Every health care worker must be prepared to recognize the symptoms of angina pectoris, as well as those of coronary insufficiency of any type.

Angina pectoris doesn't actually mean "pain": it refers to a sense of "smothering" localized in the front of the chest. It was first described by the English physician William Heberden back in the 18th century. Long before electrocardiograms or x-rays or modern pathology, Heberden deduced that this discomfort came from the heart. His younger colleague, Edward Jenner, wrote to him describing an autopsy he had carried out on a victim of angina at Bath. Jenner noted a "white, fleshy protuberance" blocking a coronary artery and guessed that this was the cause of the angina. (Jenner also discovered the smallpox vaccination, thereby saving more lives than anyone in the history of the human race.)

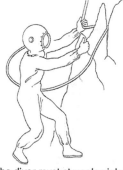

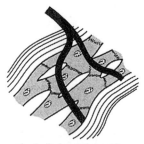

a.

If the diver must struggle violently, he will have to breathe hard, since his body needs more oxygen. The pinched air hose limits his supply of air. He begins to feel suffocated, and tugs on the air hose to warn those on the surface of his trouble.

The patient climbs stairs, walks up a hill, or eats a big meal. His heart is forced to beat faster and work harder, and the heart muscle needs more blood for the extra work. The heart muscle depends upon a narrowed, diseased coronary artery for its blood supply. It will not receive the extra blood it needs for the extra workload. The patient will usually feel pain or some other type of discomfort. It is the body's way of telling him that some area of heart muscle is not receiving enough blood.

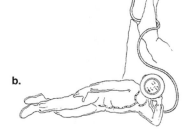

b.

The oxygen supply falls below the danger point. The diver falls into a coma. He is in danger of dying, but he is not dead yet. If the hose frees and he receives more oxygen, he can still recover.

Blood flow to an area of heart muscle falls below the amount needed to keep the cells alive. The cells are damaged, but they are not dead yet. If the blood flow increases, the cells can still recover. They can also recover if they need less blood, that is, if the heart is put at rest.

FIGURE 8–5
Angina pectoris.

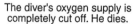

The diver's oxygen supply is completely cut off. He dies.

Blood flow to an area of heart muscle is completely cut off. The heart muscle dies. When tissue in any part of the body dies because its blood supply is cut off through blocking or hemorrhage of a terminal artery, the dead area is called an infarct.

FIGURE 8–6
Myocardial infarction—death of the heart muscle.

TABLE 8–1 How to Recognize Coronary Pain	
Characteristics of coronary pain	**How to tell if the pain is *not* coronary**
Location: anywhere in the upper half of the body; most common sites: left front of the chest, left shoulder or arm, neck (front, either side); least common sites: right front of the chest, shoulder blades.	Coronary pain never comes and goes with breathing: that is, it is never pleuritic. If pain is made worse by breathing and if it disappears when the patient holds his or her breath, it is clearly not coronary.
Causes: anginal pain, almost always brought on by physical exertion—straining, lifting, working with arms over head is especially likely to produce pain. The discomfort is always relieved by rest Prinzmetal angina: no relation to exertion; often wakens patient from sleep. Myocardial infarction: often no precipitating cause. Half of all infarctions occur during sleep. Abrupt heavy exertion, especially isometric straining, triggers the attack in about 5% of cases.	Coronary pain is never affected by coughing. If the patient says that "it hurts to cough," the pain is not coronary.
Character of pain: sense of pressure, heaviness, crushing, or aching, often accompanied by apprehension. If typical angina is present the patient will *always* stop activity at once. With infarction, the patient may become agitated and move about.	Coronary pain is not affected by motion of the arms or trunk. If the discomfort is reproduced by moving the arms or shoulders or by flexing the neck, it is not coronary.
Unusual types of discomfort: these include sudden, severe dyspnea; burning or throbbing sensations in the head, neck, or chest; sense of "pounding" of the heart; sense of dread.	Coronary pain is never brief or "stabbing." If the patient says that the pain is "quick, like a stab with a knife" and then is instantly gone, it is not coronary.

Here are the symptoms of anginal pain to look out for (Table 8–1):

- Most common and most specific: a sense of pressure anywhere in the front of the chest, often radiating up into the neck. The pain may be low in the chest, below the end of the sternum, or actually in the upper abdomen—that's why it's often mistaken for indigestion.
- The next most common site of pain is the arms: most often the left arm, sometimes both arms, rarely just the right.
- Unusual locations: I have seen several patients with well-documented anginal pain localized under the left shoulder blade. In another, the pain was localized in the left wrist. It's safe to say that pain anywhere in the upper half of the body that comes on with exertion and is relieved by rest should be considered angina until proved otherwise.
- Character of pain: Most patients think of pain as the sensation you feel when you're stabbed with a knife or stuck with a pin. It's important to explain that these are not the sensations you're talking about when you ask about heart pain. It's common to hear a patient say "I don't feel pain, just a heavy sensation in my chest." At this point an experienced cardiologist will always interrupt and explain that this "heavy sensation" is a common form of heart pain.
- "Heaviness," "pressure," or "fullness in the chest" are the most common terms used to describe angina, but they are by no means the only ones. "Tingling and burning," "a feeling as if my heart's too big for my chest," "sudden, severe anxiety," "fullness and pounding in the head and neck," and "an aching feeling, like I've pulled a muscle" are all symptoms recorded during angina pectoris. The

insufficient blood supply may interfere with the pumping action of the heart. As a result, the patient may simply become very short of breath.

One more time: The common denominator of all symptoms of the classic, typical form of angina pectoris is that the symptoms come on with exertion and are relieved by rest. Exertion like what? Exertion like walking, climbing stairs, or lifting or carrying loads, for instance. Isometric stress, or straining against a heavy weight, is especially dangerous. That's why snow shoveling often brings on coronary pain. A large meal is a type of exertion most people overlook, but it can be important. A large meal throws about the same load on the heart as walking up three flights of stairs. King Henry VIII was said to have died of a "surfeit of lampreys." In fact, he overstuffed the royal gullet and had a heart attack. Sudden emotional stress can cause the blood pressure to rise and the heart to beat faster. Angina can result.

Prinzmetal Angina

Myron Prinzmetal, an American cardiologist, described another type of angina, commonly known as the "intern's nightmare." It doesn't fit any logical pattern. The pain often comes on at rest, even though the patient doesn't feel any discomfort during exercise. It may waken patients during the early morning hours. This kind of angina is usually caused by spasm or constriction of a coronary artery. Sometimes it happens in diseased arteries, but it can also take place in completely normal vessels. Fortunately, this type of angina is rare, and it can usually be diagnosed by changes in the electrocardiogram (Fig. 8–7).

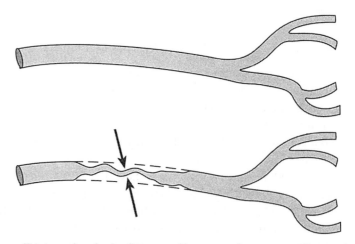

This type of angina is often caused by spasm of a coronary artery. Sometimes there is an atheroma present, but often the artery is anatomically normal.

ECG recorded during an episode of Prinzmetal angina. Note the very striking ST elevation. This was completely gone within five minutes.

FIGURE 8–7

Prinzmetal angina.

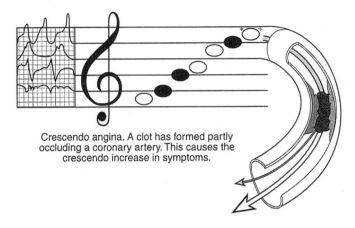

Crescendo angina. A clot has formed partly
occluding a coronary artery. This causes the
crescendo increase in symptoms.

FIGURE 8–8

Crescendo angina. A clot has formed, partly occluding a coronary
artery. This causes the crescendo increase in symptoms.

Crescendo Angina: Coronary Insufficiency

When a musical score reads "crescendo," it means "play louder and louder, progressively." That's a good description of this dangerous type of angina. The pain comes on more often, or it's more severe, or it comes on with less effort—sometimes all three. In an especially dangerous form of crescendo angina, the pain comes on at rest or wakens the patient from sleep, especially in the early morning hours. It's now clear that when this happens a blood clot has started to form at the diseased, narrowed spot in the artery. The clot doesn't block the artery completely, but it cuts down flow below the danger point and there is the beginning of damage to the heart muscle (Fig. 8–8). Complete closure and sudden death are immediate risks. The patient with crescendo angina must be put in a hospital at once. The pain may last longer than in typical angina—sometimes as long as 30 minutes. The term **coronary insufficiency** is often used in these cases. Again, the combination of a clot and an atheroma is responsible and the risk is the same as in crescendo angina. Note the predicament of the diver in Figure 8–5 and you'll have a good idea of what goes on in crescendo angina and coronary insufficiency.

Myocardial Infarction

This is the full-blown "heart attack." The word **infarct** means that an area of tissue has died because its blood supply has been cut off. Myocardial infarction means that an area of heart muscle has died because a coronary artery has been completely blocked. It is now certain that this happens because of a blood clot that forms in a diseased, narrowed part of a coronary artery. The word for clot is **thrombus,** hence the common term "coronary thrombosis."

Note our unlucky diver in Figure 8–6. The most common symptom of myocardial infarction is pain, often exactly like the pain of angina pectoris, except that it doesn't go away. The pain of infarction can be so severe the victim can hardly stand it, or it may be so mild that it's passed off as heartburn or neuralgia. In Framingham, Massachusetts, a large number of autopsy records were examined. To everyone's surprise, 25% of the patients whose hearts showed the scars of infarcts had no medical history of any kind. In other words, about a quarter of all infarcts are "silent." The victim never knows they happened.

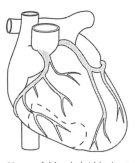

1hour : A blood clot blocks a diseased artery. There is some injury to the muscle almost at once.

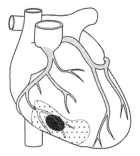

12–24 hours: A central core of tissue is dead. There is a zone of injured tissue that is still alive and can be saved.

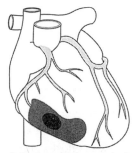

5–21 days: All the marginal tissues either die or recover. The infarct is now a solid mass of decaying and healing tissue.

8 weeks: A firm scar has formed. Healing is complete.

FIGURE 8–9

Sequence of events of myocardial infarction.

FIGURE 8–10

Ventricular fibrillation. At the onset, the complexes are larger and more nearly regular. At the end, however, the tracing dwindles into the typical nondescript deflections produced by ventricular fibrillation.

What happens to the heart muscle in an infarct? Figure 8–9 explains the sequence of events.

What's the risk of myocardial infarction? It's high. Fifty percent of people who suffer a myocardial infarct die on the spot before medical aid can be summoned. Once the patient reaches the hospital, on the other hand, the risk is very small: the risk of dying of a first heart attack in a properly staffed coronary care unit with conservative medical management is only 7%.

Why do people die after a myocardial infarct? First, the heart may stop its regular beating and go into a fast, feeble twitching, called ventricular fibrillation. The patient drops as if shot, and death follows within 10 minutes (Fig. 8–10).

Second, the amount of muscle destroyed may be large enough to weaken the pumping action of the heart: congestive heart failure follows. If 30% or more of the muscle

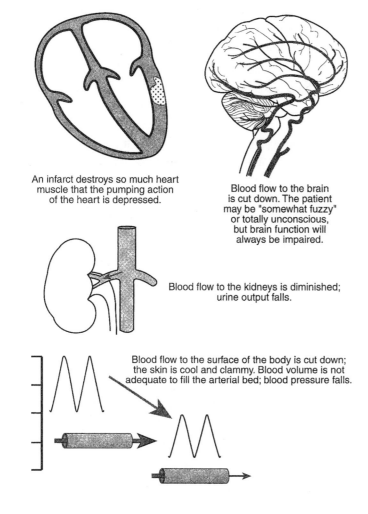

An infarct destroys so much heart muscle that the pumping action of the heart is depressed.

Blood flow to the brain is cut down. The patient may be "somewhat fuzzy" or totally unconscious, but brain function will always be impaired.

Blood flow to the kidneys is diminished; urine output falls.

Blood flow to the surface of the body is cut down; the skin is cool and clammy. Blood volume is not adequate to fill the arterial bed; blood pressure falls.

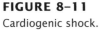

FIGURE 8–11
Cardiogenic shock.

mass of the left ventricle is destroyed, there won't be enough pump to sustain life and the patient will die. Third, the patient may go into cardiogenic shock—this is usually fatal.

What is shock? This is one of the most important definitions for any health worker to have firmly in mind. Shock has nothing to do with coming home and finding your house on fire. The medical definition of shock is simple: **there isn't enough blood circulating through the tissues of the body to keep them functioning**.

The simplest kind of shock to understand comes from hemorrhage: someone loses a great deal of blood quickly and there isn't enough left to support the needs of the body.

There are more complicated causes of shock. Overwhelming infection may produce shock by shunting blood into internal reservoirs where it can't be used. This is called septic shock.

Cardiogenic shock results from a massive myocardial infarct that destroys so much ventricular tissue that there isn't enough forward flow out of the heart to support the rest of the body (Fig. 8–11). This inadequate blood flow produces changes in the function of four key areas of the body. These changes are easy to detect and the physician can usually establish the diagnosis within minutes.

Cardiogenic shock is very dangerous. The mortality has traditionally been about 80%. Modern means of treatment have improved the outlook somewhat, but the grim fact remains that cardiogenic shock is fatal more often than not.

THE DIAGNOSIS OF CORONARY ARTERY DISEASE

If coronary artery disease doesn't produce symptoms, it probably won't be detected. Actually, the word *symptoms* is misleading: it should be *symptom* because there's only one. Painful discomfort of some type is the only symptom of coronary artery disease in the vast majority of cases. It's usually the only warning the patient gets.

What the discomfort feels like, where the patient feels it, what brings it on, and what relieves it are, in a real sense, life-and-death questions since the answers will often establish the presence of coronary artery disease with an accuracy approaching 100%.

The physician may not be the one asking these questions: nurses, paramedics, technicians, and office receptionists will often be the first to hear the patient's story. An intelligent, informed listener is in a position to save health and life.

Diagnosis of Angina Pectoris

A reliable, carefully elicited history of typical anginal pain is about 90% accurate in establishing the presence of coronary artery disease. The electrocardiogram may be normal or may show some nonspecific changes. If the electrocardiogram is recorded during anginal pain, it will usually show an injury current—an electric potential that comes from injured heart muscle (Fig. 8–12).

It's impossible to follow a patient around with an electrocardiograph all day, but it is possible to produce angina under controlled conditions and record an electrocardiogram at the same time. This is the goal of exercise stress testing. The patient exercises on a treadmill or other machine and the electrocardiogram is recorded during the procedure (see Chap. 11).

Exercise testing can be carried out using radioactive tracers. When heart muscle is not getting enough blood, it will not pick up the isotope thallium. The patient exercises until pain appears or an injury current shows up on the electrocardiogram. At this point, the isotope is injected. The healthy muscle will pick up the isotope, but there will be a blank spot in the area with inadequate blood flow. This blank spot will fill in after a rest period when the blood flow comes back to normal, thereby making it clear that the conditions of angina pectoris were present (Fig. 8–13).

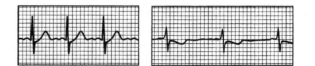

FIGURE 8–12

There's a normal ECG strip on the left. In the strip on the right you see depression of the segment that comes after the verticular spike and before the T wave. This is caused by an *injury* current that arises from heart muscle that isn't getting enough blood.

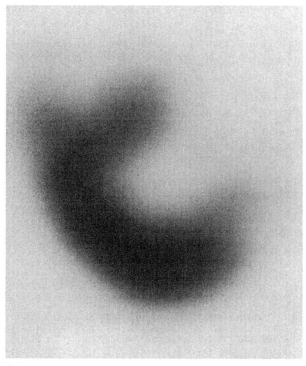
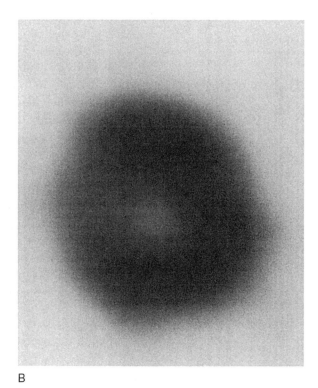

A   B

FIGURE 8–13

Demonstration of reversible ischemia in the myocardium with the use of radioactive thallium. The views are taken from the front. **A.** The recording is made just after treadmill exercise. There is a large white area beginning in the center and directed upward and to the right that indicates no radioactivity. In other words, there is heart muscle that is temporarily nonfunctioning: it cannot pick up the radioactive material. **B.** After a rest period, the whole heart is outlined by the radioactivity: the heart muscle that was temporarily ischemic is now perfused normally with blood. This is a very accurate demonstration of transient myocardial ischemia, or angina. (Courtesy of Dr. James Woolfenden, University of Arizona Medical Center.)

Diagnosis of Crescendo Angina

Everyone who has coronary artery disease should know a great deal about crescendo angina. Unfortunately, most patients don't even know what it is.

You've just read about the classic symptoms of anginal pain that you find in every textbook. Next comes an important and very practical question: *Is painful discomfort the only symptom when an area of heart muscle isn't getting enough blood?*

Now that stress testing is available, we've learned more about what the patient actually feels when an area of heart muscle is deprived of an adequate blood supply. The term "anginal equivalent" describes symptoms *other than pain* that tell you some heart muscle isn't getting enough blood.

When Heberden made the epochal discovery that a certain type of painful discomfort was associated with coronary artery disease, he did it just by good clinical observation. All he had to go by were the patient's symptoms—no electrocardiogram, no isotopes, no echocardiograms; in other words, he had no way of actually demonstrating that there was inadequate blood flow to some area of heart muscle. He could only assume that was happening because the patient felt painful discomfort. As a result, for centuries everyone assumed that painful discomfort was the only symptom of the disease.

Now we can actually demonstrate inadequate blood flow by several types of stress testing. As a result, it's possible to learn more about the symptoms of this disorder because we can record the symptoms while the patient is walking on a treadmill or being subjected to chemical stress.

In the early days of monitored stress testing, my colleagues and I carried out a simple study on a number of patients with known coronary artery disease.

We put 186 patients with known coronary artery disease on a treadmill and watched their electrocardiogram on an oscilloscope.

When an injury current appeared, we asked them what they were feeling. The results were surprising. (The injury current in the electrocardiogram is an actual electric potential that's produced when heart muscle is injured by inadequate blood supply. See Fig. 8–12.)

We found that the commonest symptom was severe, sometimes frightening shortness of breath (dyspnea).

The second commonest was shortness of breath followed by pain.

Third was a set of vague distressing symptoms, such as severe apprehension, a sense that the whole chest "felt strange," and others.

Fourth was typical anginal pain alone.

Finally, in almost 11% of patients there were no symptoms at all. The ischemia was "silent."

This study was published in a medical journal in 1968 [1] and in the last year it was rediscovered by an eminent Israeli cardiologist, Dr. Shlomo Stern[2], who has revived interest in the whole subject of dyspnea as a manifestation of ischemia.

The reason for the dyspnea in these patients is simple. When heart muscle isn't getting enough blood it "stiffens"—it loses elasticity or, as cardiologists like to say, it loses compliance. It isn't elastic enough to handle the inflow of blood from the lungs and there's a "backup" of pressure into the pulmonary vessels within a few heartbeats. Of course, shortness of breath follows within seconds.

Moral: *Severe, abrupt dyspnea, out of proportion to physical activity, is very often a marker of inadequate blood flow to a region of myocardium. The examiner searching for coronary artery disease should always ask about shortness of breath that comes on abruptly, with exertion. Sudden severe shortness of breath before or during pain makes it much more likely that the pain is anginal.*

Stress echocardiography means that an echocardiogram is recorded before treadmill exercise and immediately after. Changes in motion of the heart muscle or abnormalities of contraction are a very reliable sign of coronary insufficiency (see Chap. 24). Stress echocardiography is simpler and cheaper than isotope testing and both methods are much more accurate than simple electrocardiographic stress testing.

Therefore, if a physician is trying to find out whether coronary artery disease is present or not, one of these two methods should be used.

Simple electrocardiographic stress testing, on the other hand, is useful to quantitate the significance of known coronary disease. (For example, how much exercise does it take to bring on angina? What is it safe for the patient to do?)

If a patient cannot walk enough to carry out a stress test, chemical stressing can be used with Persantine or dobutamine. These impose a stress similar to exercise but there are some hazards and they should be used with caution and only when the patient cannot walk enough to carry on a treadmill stress test.

The reason patients need to know about crescendo angina is that the patient is in the best position to make the diagnosis.

Right after the patient comes the office receptionist, who will hear the symptoms over the phone, or the nurse in the emergency room, or the technician or paramedic encountering the patient in a variety of settings. In other words, crescendo angina is a diagnosis based entirely on symptoms.

Here are the phrases that should flash a red light: "I'm having more heart pain," "It comes on easier than it used to, and I can't walk as far before it starts to hurt," "I have had to take more nitroglycerin tablets these last few days," and so on. Anyone talking to a patient known to have angina pectoris should always ask the patient about nitroglycerin: Taking more tablets lately? How many more? For how long? If the patient needs nitroglycerin more times per day, or needs it after less effort, or if it takes more tablets to relieve the pain, the diagnosis of crescendo angina is established.

Most important of all are these two questions: "Does the pain come on at rest?" and "Does the pain waken you from sleep?" If the answer to either question is yes, the most dangerous type of crescendo angina is present and immediate hospitalization is essential.

There's no red light that starts flashing on the patient's chest that says "Alert! Crescendo!" What is there, for anyone with clinical ears to hear, is an unmistakable set of symptoms. **Crescendo angina is a medical emergency**. Any patient who describes crescendo angina must be hospitalized at once in an intensive care unit. There may or may not be changes in the ECG: the symptoms are all the evidence needed to establish the diagnosis. Every attempt should be made to record an ECG during pain, because this may give powerful confirmation and help with decisions about treatment.

Coronary Arteriography

This is the gold standard for detecting coronary artery disease in any stage. A catheter is threaded up an artery and into the heart. Dye is injected directly into the coronary arteries, and x-ray movies, called cineangiograms, are recorded (Fig. 8–14). Even very small abnormalities can be detected, and it is also possible to get an accurate idea of the pumping efficiency of the heart.

Diagnosis of Myocardial Infarction

When the pain of myocardial infarction is typical, it's obvious to anyone with minimal health care training. When the pain isn't typical, it gives physicians nightmares. Read again the description of anginal pain and observe this rule: **When pain of this kind lasts 30 minutes or more, there's a myocardial infarct until you prove there isn't**.

Electrocardiogram

At least 75% of the time there will be changes in the electrocardiogram (see Chap. 11). Sometimes they are so typical that the physician can be certain that an infarction is in progress and can be reasonably sure of the vessel involved. Sometimes changes are minor and nonspecific. In possibly 10% of cases the electrocardiogram will be normal in the early stages of the infarction.

Blood Tests

Certain chemicals, or enzymes, are released into the blood by infarcted tissue. Creatine phosphokinase, or CPK, is released from injured heart muscle as well as from other types of tissue. The specific part of CPK released from heart muscle is referred to as the MB band. A rise in MB-CPK to abnormal levels is almost 100% specific for myocardial infarction. Unfortunately, it takes about 12 hours for these abnormal blood levels to appear.

Happily, a new rapid blood test has been developed that assists in early diagnosis of myocardial infarction. A form of myoglobin is detected in the blood following infarction,

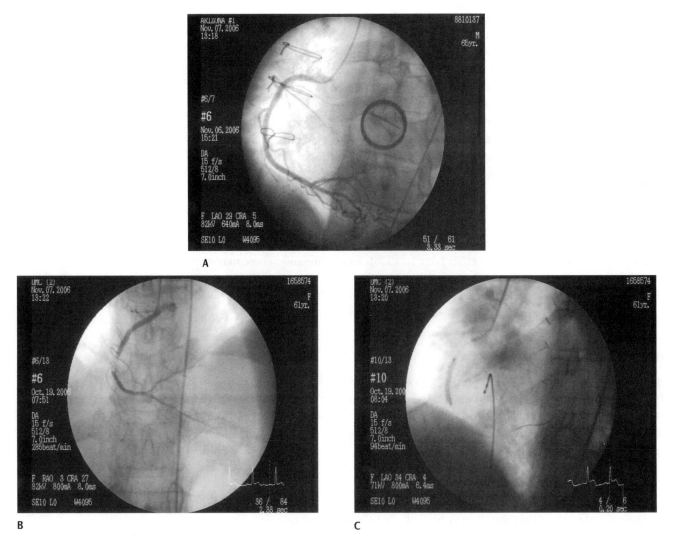

FIGURE 8–14

A. Angiogram showing a normal right coronary artery. There are also sternal wires from previous cardiac surgery and a St. Jude mitral valve (on the right). **B.** Angiogram of a diseased right coronary artery. The area that doesn't fill with die represents a lesion that almost occludes the artery. **C.** Introduction of a ballon catheter to dilate the narrowed area. **D.** Excellent result after angioplasty with open coronary artery and no visible lesion. (Courtesy of Dr. Karl B. Kern, University of Arizona Medical Center.)

and it appears within 2 hours. This is a one-way correlation. A normal myoglobin 2 hours after the onset of symptoms absolutely rules out myocardial infarction. On the other hand, a rise in myoglobin means only that an infract *may* be present. It's not an absolute diagnosis: many other causes can produce a rise in myoglobin.

Troponin fragments are amazingly sensitive for myocardial necrosis (cell death) of any size. The problem is that severe angina (crescendo or sustained) will very often produce very small areas of necrosis without an actual infarct. Troponin fragments are so sensitive that they'll rise in response to these micronecrotic areas caused by angina when there isn't an actual infarct.

Rises in troponin also occur with severe kidney disease. *However, a normal troponin absolutely rules out myocardial infarction.*

Some years ago I served on the Peer Review Committees of the American College of Cardiology, and we agonized for months over the criteria needed to justify admission to

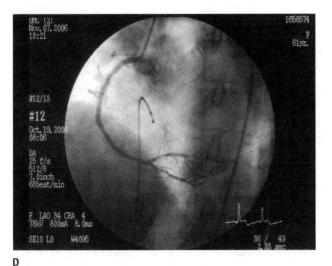

D

FIGURE 8–14 *(continued)*

a hospital with a diagnosis of possible myocardial infarction. Since the blood tests *may* not turn positive for 12 hours and the electrocardiogram may be normal in the early stages, there remains only one criterion: **Discomfort that arouses suspicion of a myocardial infarct plus a rise in troponin or myoglobin is all the physician has to go on in many cases and these findings alone are enough to warrant admission to the hospital for initial care and further testing**.

In other words, all the electronic space age technology in the world doesn't compare with intelligent questioning by an experienced physician when it comes to the early diagnosis of this most common of cardiac disasters.

By the same token, this criterion means that a significant number of patients will "rule out"—that is, blood tests and electrocardiograms will remain normal and it will appear that the pain was caused by something else. This has to be accepted at this stage of medical science. It's like making the meshes on a net small enough to be sure you catch all the barracudas: you will also catch some harmless perch, but that can't be avoided. A competent, conscientious cardiologist will find that about 25% of the patients admitted with suspicion of a myocardial infarct won't have one; it will turn out that the pain was caused by irritation in the lower esophagus or in the chest wall itself. If the number isn't that high, the cardiologist isn't being careful enough, and some infarcts are going to be missed.

TREATMENT OF CORONARY ARTERY DISEASE

There is no way of "dissolving" an atheroma in a coronary artery by medical means. There are no medications or drugs that can "shrink" an atheroma or make it disappear, contrary to the claims of quacks. Medical science simply hasn't progressed that far yet. Treatment has four bases:

1. Medical management. It's possible to lower the oxygen requirements of the heart muscle, and thus balance supply and demand. In some cases, it's also possible to use medication to dilate the coronary arteries temporarily.

2. Surgical bypass procedures. A healthy artery or vein from another part of the body can be used to create a "detour" around the diseased area.

3. The diseased artery can sometimes be opened by means of a balloon attached to a catheter. Laser beams can open a small hole in an atheroma and a catheter with a special small, high-speed rotating blade can actually remove most of the lesion. Fine-mesh wire sleeves, or stents, can be inserted by catheter to hold the vessel open after the lesion has been removed. None of these methods are perfect, and there is still a high reclosure rate—as much as 30%. This reclosure of the vessel is known as **restenosis**.

4. Treatment depends first of all on the clinical presentation of the disease. Start with angina pectoris.

MEDICAL MANAGEMENT OF ANGINA PECTORIS

1. Lower the oxygen requirements of the heart muscle by:

   a. limiting physical exertion

   b. controlling blood pressure

   c. using beta-blocking drugs

2. Increase coronary blood flow or lower the work of the heart by nitrates (nitroglycerin and isosorbide). Use nitroglycerin prophylactically (before exercise, etc.).

3. Lower blood pressure and possibly dilate coronary arteries with calcium-blocking drugs.

4. Prevent more atheroma formation by lowering blood lipids through diet and medication, if needed.

   Note: Treatment of angina pectoris is based primarily on lowering the oxygen requirements of the heart muscle to balance the inadequate blood flow. It is also possible, in some cases, to increase blood flow through the coronary arteries temporarily. In addition, the patient's style of living can be changed to avoid demands that exceed the limited coronary supply.

Details About Drugs

The medical use of nitroglycerin began with an observation by an astute French physician during the siege of Paris in the Franco-Prussian War. He noticed that workers handling dynamite became flushed and complained of headaches, and he reasoned, correctly, that inhaling the fumes of nitroglycerin caused blood vessels to dilate. By this time in medical history, everybody knew that angina pectoris was caused by inadequate blood flow to an area of heart muscle. Simple logic suggested the use of nitroglycerin to dilate arteries. It worked dramatically, and nitroglycerin remains the cornerstone of treatment of angina pectoris to this day.

Nitroglycerin has two beneficial effects. First, it dilates the veins of the entire body, thus holding back a large flow of blood from the heart and "unloading" the heart muscle. The oxygen requirements of the heart muscle fall dramatically; supply and demand of blood flow are back in balance within seconds.

Second, in some cases, nitroglycerin actually dilates the coronary arteries. This effect has been much debated, but studies during cardiac catheterization leave no question that it does happen. The coronary arteries can be shown to expand, with an increase in blood flow during peak effect of nitroglycerin. Dilation of diseased arteries isn't always possible: when a mass of calcified hard fat is plugging up great parts of an artery it can't expand any more than an iron pipe can. However, when arteries are less severely diseased, they can react to nitroglycerin, and healthy arteries can expand substantially with increased blood flow to the threatened area.

Sublingual nitroglycerin with rapid absorption from a tablet placed under the tongue is unquestionably effective. It should be used to relieve any anginal pain. In addition, it should be used prophylactically. This is an effect too often overlooked by clinicians.

When nitroglycerin is taken before exertion, it can prevent the anginal reaction. As an example, I recently observed a patient during treadmill testing when pain and ECG change appeared after 2 minutes of moderate exertion. One tablet of sublingual nitroglycerin was administered and allowed to take effect. Subsequently, the patient walked 15 minutes through a full treadmill test without pain and without change in the electrocardiogram. Any patient with angina should be thoroughly trained in the prophylactic use of the drug. The patient should always be instructed to take nitroglycerin before any activity that might be expected to bring on an attack.

Long-acting nitrolgycerin can be administered by patch worn on the skin or by capsules or tablets that are swallowed. Sometimes these dosage forms are effective, but they wear off quickly as the patient develops tolerance to the drug. By giving the drugs intermittently, with "rest periods," this loss of potency can be avoided or minimized. It is now known that the nitrates work by releasing nitric oxide from the cells in the lining of the blood vessels, both arteries and veins. Nitric oxide dilates the vessels, but there's only a certain amount available: when it's used up, the drug has no effect. That's why it's essential to have rest periods—so that cells can recharge their nitric oxide content.

Isosorbide dinitrate is a related drug that releases nitric oxide and dilates veins: its action is longer—about 2 hours. After that, the cells lining the blood vessels need time to regenerate their load of nitric oxide. If isosorbide dinitrate is given four times a day, that equals about 8 hours of helpful dilation of blood vessels—not a bad yield, and often life-saving. Again, patients develop tolerance and the drug loses its effect: intermittent dosing with rest periods is essential.

Beta-blocking drugs have been important for the treatment of angina pectoris. Remember that in treatment of hypertension, these drugs work by blocking certain effects of the adrenalinelike substances that occur normally in the body. When these substances are blocked, the heart becomes a slower, more efficient pump and uses less blood, for any given level of work. Unfortunately there are times when these drugs can't be used. If the patient suffers from asthma or peripheral vascular disease they are dangerous. Otherwise, they should always be used in the treatment of coronary artery disease. Formerly it was thought that they could not be used in the setting of congestive heart failure but this notion has been discarded. Beta blockers must be employed cautiously with slow progression of dosage if heart failure is present, but they are extremely helpful in this setting (see Chap. 17).

The same calcium-blocking drugs used in the treatment of hypertension are helpful in treatment of angina pectoris. Since these drugs dilate arteries, it is believed that they may dilate some part of the coronary circulation. In addition, they lower blood pressure, thereby helping to keep down the oxygen requirements of the heart muscle. The effect of calcium blockers is not as dramatic or as well documented as that of the beta blockers, but they are unquestionably valuable, especially in combination with nitrates and beta blockers (Fig. 8–15).

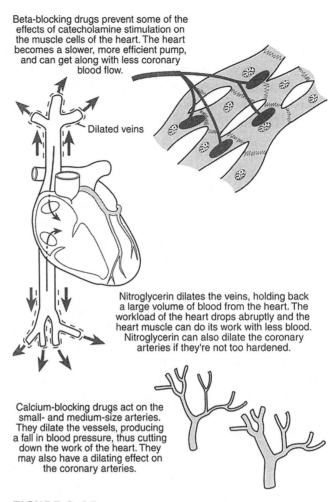

Beta-blocking drugs prevent some of the effects of catecholamine stimulation on the muscle cells of the heart. The heart becomes a slower, more efficient pump, and can get along with less coronary blood flow.

Dilated veins

Nitroglycerin dilates the veins, holding back a large volume of blood from the heart. The workload of the heart drops abruptly and the heart muscle can do its work with less blood. Nitroglycerin can also dilate the coronary arteries if they're not too hardened.

Calcium-blocking drugs act on the small- and medium-size arteries. They dilate the vessels, producing a fall in blood pressure, thus cutting down the work of the heart. They may also have a dilating effect on the coronary arteries.

FIGURE 8–15
Medical management of angina pectoris.

TREATMENT OF CRESCENDO ANGINA

1. Bedrest in a coronary care unit.
2. Blood and ECG tests to rule out myocardial infarction.
3. Intravenous heparin. It is now known that in the majority of cases a thrombus has formed and is partly occluding the diseased artery. These clots are usually "white clots" formed by masses of platelets; heparin and aspirin specifically control and eradicate platelet clots. Unless there is some reason that aspirin shouldn't be administered (e.g., a bleeding ulcer), it should always be started together with the heparin.
4. Maximal medical management with nitroglycerin or other nitrates, beta blockers, and possibly calcium blockers.
5. In most cases the symptoms will subside. After a "cooling-off" period, coronary arteriograms should be recorded if the patient is a candidate for angioplasty (Fig. 8–14) or bypass surgery. If the patient is too old or too sick with complicating diseases to tolerate either of these procedures, intensive medical management should be continued. Prolonged use of an anticoagulant

(Coumadin) may be useful in this group of patients, although the evidence is questionable.

Why should a patient be catheterized after an episode of crescendo angina? Simple. The syndrome makes it clear that there's a coronary artery very close to total occlusion but not closed yet. If the vessel closes, the patient faces a 50% risk that goes with any myocardial infarction. If catheterization shows that the vessel or vessels can be opened or bypassed, and if the patient is a reasonable candidate for these procedures, the whole process may be literally lifesaving.

Every available study, however, has made it clear that the cardiologist shouldn't rush in to do the catheterization as soon as the diagnosis has been made. It's clear that patients do better after a cooling-off period with maximal medical management, probably because the myocardium has stabilized in electrical and metabolic terms. On the other hand, if the symptoms persist in spite of intensive medical treatment there is no choice: catheterization with coronary arteriography becomes an emergency procedure.

TREATMENT OF MYOCARDIAL INFARCTION

When I was an intern in the eventful winter of 1941–1942, myocardial infarcts were treated with 8 weeks of bedrest, oxygen, and morphine for pain. There was nothing else to do, apart from treating such complications as congestive failure and shock. Now we know that prolonged bedrest isn't necessary. Most patients with uncomplicated myocardial infarcts can go home in a week. Medical management of myocardial infarction begins with maximal possible "rest" for the heart. The workload of the heart depends on two things: heart rate and blood pressure. The slower the heart rate and the lower the blood pressure, the less workload there is on the heart. Therefore, the first step in medical management is a combination of bedrest and medication to produce the slowest heart rate and the lowest blood pressure the patient can tolerate. Early orders should always include:

1. **Bedrest** or rest in a "cardiac" or reclining chair.
2. **Relief of pain with morphine**. Morphine is an excellent drug at this stage of infarction. In addition to relieving pain, it causes a fall in the levels of dangerous adrenalinelike substances or catecholamine that usually rise abruptly at the time of infarction. It also dilates the veins gently, thereby "unloading" the heart.
3. **Control of blood pressure**. If the pressure is elevated it should always be lowered carefully, in steps, with nitroprusside.
4. **Small meals**. This is often overlooked, but a large meal is as much work for the heart as walking up three flights of stairs. Blood flow through large arteries such as the one to the liver increases as much as 30% after a large meal. (When Dr. Master introduced the Carrel diet of four glasses of milk a day, he produced the first significant drop in mortality from infarction in the New York hospitals where it was employed.)
5. **Beta-blocking drugs**. By producing a slower, more efficient heartbeat these drugs are so effective that they should always be administered if the heart rate permits.

Other routine measures include:

6. **Oxygen**. Even though blood oxygen levels may be normal, oxygen is always given to the patient to enhance oxygen delivery at the cellular level in the infarcted area.

7. **Aspirin**. The benefit of aspirin in infarction is substantial. It should always be administered early.

8. **ACE inhibitors.** These should always be added to the medical regimen before the patient is discharged.

These are routine measures that are remarkably effective in lowering the incidence of mortality from myocardial infarction.

Two new dramatic developments have changed the management of myocardial infarction drastically.

- **Thrombolytic agents.** For more than 10 years agents have been available to dissolve the clot that is almost always associated with myocardial infarction. The two agents now in use are **streptokinase** and **TPA (tissue plasminogen activator).** When either is administered *early* in the course of infarction, the clot can be dissolved and normal blood flow is restored.

- **"Early" means within 4 hours**. There may be some benefit up to 6 hours, but after that it's too late: the myocardial cells in the infarcted area die and no amount of new blood will bring them back. Furthermore, it's risky to send a rush of blood through an area of dead tissue; it can cause dangerous arrhythmias. Some investigators have claimed benefit up to 24 hours after infarction, but the consensus is that 6 hours is about the outer limit for thrombolytic drugs.

Thrombolytic agents presented the medical profession with a new form of human biology—the **post-thrombolytic infarct**. After the clot, what? There are three possible courses of action.

1. Catheterize the patient at once and try to correct the diseased artery with angioplasty or surgery.

2. Wait a week or so and then proceed with catheterization and possible correction.

3. Wait to see if the patient has more pain (angina) or a second infarct. If the patient has no more symptoms or findings, treat medically. If more pain appears or if the patient has suspicious findings during exercise testing after healing is complete, go ahead with catheterization and correction.

Thanks to two large studies on thousands of patients, there's no longer any question about the best course. The TIMI (Thrombolysis in Myocardial Infarction) IIa study in the United States and the SWIFT (Should We Intervene Following Thrombolysis) study in Europe have tested the three possible courses, and the results were published in leading heart journals in the spring of 1990. The answers are simple and straightforward.

Option 1 should never be used: there's a higher complication rate and probably a higher mortality. Options 2 and 3 give exactly the same results: the mortality in the hospital and 1 year later are the same. Function of the heart is the same after 1 year. The 3-year follow-up studies published in 1994 strongly supported the conservative option (option 3). At the end of 3 years, the patients were compared in terms of survival, cardiac complications, and cardiac function. Option 3 gave results identical with option 2 and better than option 1. In other words, routine catheterization following thrombolysis, whether immediate or delayed, provides no benefit and is not justified.

There's one enormous advantage to option 3: it saves money spent on unnecessary catheterizations. Under option 3 only those patients with more pain following the infarct or with a poor treadmill performance are catheterized. It turned out these were exactly the patients who should have been catheterized: some 85% of them had lesions in the coronary arteries that needed correcting and were correctable. If all patients are catheterized (option 2), 75% of the procedures may be unnecessary. Take a hard look at option 3. It's the only protocol justified by current cardiovascular research.

One exception: a patient in cardiogenic shock after a myocardial infarct who doesn't respond to medical management may benefit from catheterization and correction of the coronary artery disease. Results so far in this group are only suggestive.

Early Angioplasty

A number of studies have compared early catherization and balloon angioplasty with thrombolytic therapy. It now seems clear that if the patient can reach a catheterization facility within 90 minutes of the onset of symptoms, catheterization and correction of the lesion by angioplasty or other means provides good results. That's an hour and a half, and it isn't much time for the patient to recognize that the pain might be a heart attack, arrive at an emergency room, and end up in a catheterization laboratory to have the vessel opened. In fact, it's rarely possible to do all that in such a brief interval. Those 90 minutes are the "golden minutes" when heart muscle can be rescued by opening the diseased artery. After that it's probably too late. Even though that's a well-established observation, in many centers myocardial infarcts are often treated by catheterization long after the "golden period" has passed. What's the benefit at this point? That's part of the current "Great Debate."

Assuming the patient reaches medical care within 90 minutes, what's the proper course? Thrombolysis? Angioplasty? Both?

There have been many studies comparing these three approaches and the numbers are becoming clearer.

Assuming the patient reaches the catheterization facility within 90 minutes, angioplasty gives a slightly better result in terms of early death—but the difference is very slight: 1.3% to be exact. Statisticians would say that number barely reaches significance.

Reinfarction *later*, however, occurs more often after thrombolysis than after angioplasty and this, of course, gives a higher total mortality. In other words, there are more *late* complications after thrombolysis than after angioplasty.

To put the controversy very simply:

1. Thrombolysis and angioplasty give about the same early benefit.
2. Angioplasty prevents *later* complications such as reinfarction.
3. If a patient can be delivered to a catheterization facility within 90 minutes of onset of symptoms, angioplasty is the preferred solution. (In the United States today, this won't happen very often: the time is just too short.)
4. If a patient cannot reach a catheterization facility within that time, thrombolysis should be administered. (After all, it takes only a few minutes to administer a thrombolytic agent in any emergency room.)
5. If the patient has more pain or ECG change in the following hours, catheterization should be carried out at once.
6. If the patient has an uneventful course after thrombolysis, catheterization can be delayed to allow the affected tissues time to stabilize.

Should all patients who have suffered a myocardial infarct undergo catheterization? They certainly do in the United States today. The argument is that the patient has survived an infarct that carried a 50% mortality: it's common sense to see if another infarct is pending and try to prevent it. Does late catherization and intervention after an infarct prolong life? The answer is yes, but only in a minority of individuals with coronary artery disease (see below).

THE GREAT DEBATE: INVASIVE VERSUS NONINVASIVE DIAGNOSIS AND TREATMENT OF CORONARY DISEASE

Diagnosis comes first, of course.

To summarize everything that's gone before, the physician can diagnose coronary artery disease by several methods: ECG plus symptoms, stress testing, and coronary angiograms. Coronary artery disease can be treated medically, or by angioplasty or bypass surgery. Coronary angiography, angioplasty, and bypass grafting are lumped under the heading of *invasive diagnosis and treatment.*

What are the benefits of invasive diagnosis and treatment?

First, angioplasty and bypass surgery do relieve pain. As a result they make it possible for patients to live better lives, resume employment, and enjoy recreation.

Do they prolong life?

They prolong life only in a minority of coronary patients. Which patients?

First, they prolong life in patients with disease of the left main coronary artery—no question here. (Risk untreated is about 15% per year.)

Second, invasive diagnosis and treatment prolong life in patients with disease at the origin of the left anterior descending coronary artery plus depressed left ventricular function. (Risk is at least 10+% per year.)

Third, they may help patients with disease of all three coronary arteries. (Risk is about 15% per year.)

Fourth, they may possibly prolong life in patients with disease at the origin of a coronary artery that provides most of the blood supply to the myocardium. (Risk is not clear, but probably substantial.)

In all other categories of coronary disease invasive methods only relieve pain: they cannot be shown to prolong life.

What percentage of all coronary disease do these four categories comprise?

Nobody knows. You'd think someone would investigate this all-important question, but so far nobody has. Certainly these categories constitute a minority of all cases of coronary disease—possibly 30% or fewer.

How can a patient find out about personal risk?

Well, there's the rub. Catheterization with coronary arteriography is the only way to find out which arteries are hardened and to what extent. Without that knowledge there's no way to calculate the risk.

You can therefore make the argument that, in order to determine risk and thus decide whether angioplasty or bypass surgery will prolong life, catheterization is indicated in any patient when coronary artery disease is known to be present or is strongly suspected. Certainly that's the standard practice in the United States today.

On the other had, two large-scale studies of "stable" angina pectoris have been carried out in Wales and in Germany. ("Stable" angina means angina that can be produced predictably, at a given level of exertion.) Patients in each study were divided into "invasive" and "noninvasive" groups. The noninvasive patients received maximal medical management plus a vigorous, managed walking–exercise program. The invasive group underwent angiography and angioplasty or bypass surgery, as indicated.

In both the Welsh and German studies the noninvasive group did better! ("Better" means fewer deaths and fewer major cardiac events as well as better functional state.)

As I stated, standard practice in the United States today is to catheterize anyone with real evidence of coronary artery disease, with the hope of prolonging life in the minority of patients who have the severe disease types listed above. Is this the best course? We await more evidence.

PREVENTION

The best thing to do about any disease is to prevent it. To prevent a disease you usually have to know the cause, and we certainly don't know the whole cause of coronary artery disease. It's clear that there are some things anyone can do to lessen the risk of coronary artery disease and it appears a lot of people have been doing them—the death rate from coronary disease has dropped dramatically in the last 5 years.

1. Don't smoke. The risk of dying of coronary artery disease goes up 300% if you smoke.
2. Check blood fats. If they're elevated, get professional advice on diet and possibly medication to lower them. Stay with the program.
3. Eat well. Even if blood fats are normal, eat a diet that's rich in fish, fowl, vegetables, and grain and low in meat fat, dairy fat, and other sources of dangerous types of fat, like tropical oils. Get a standard, low-cholesterol, low-fat diet from any library or from the American Heart Association.
4. Control hypertension.
5. If you're overweight, lose weight. Obesity isn't a risk factor for coronary disease by itself, but it leads to high blood pressure. If you have clinical coronary disease, there's no point in carrying around a lot of useless weight.
6. Get regular, reasonable exercise. It's not clear that exercise prevents coronary disease in the first place, buts there's no question that regular exercise like walking is very beneficial in the treatment of known coronary disease. (In this sense, exercise could be listed as "secondary prevention"—that is, prevention of further extension or worsening of a disease.) "Cardiac rehabilitation" with sophisticated exercise machines and blinking lights is very popular and widely utilized in many centers. The sad fact is that this kind of organized postinfarct exercise program has not been shown to prevent death or complications and it does not prolong life. Patients state that they "feel better" and this is solemnly described as "improved quality of life," but in my own practice I simply start people on a walking program with reasonable increases in distance every week. No expense, same results.
7. Reduce mental stress. No clear data here, but there's no question that anybody functions better and feels better generally if periods of relaxation and diversion are part of every day, week, and month. You may have read a great deal about Type A personalities and coronary disease, but the data are wildly contradictory and there are no scientifically acceptable conclusions yet. In fact, some psychologists have questioned whether there is such a thing as a Type A personality, while others have claimed that Type A individuals have less rather than more coronary artery disease!

Note: The newest studies suggest that very strenuous lowering of blood fats actually makes the atheromas get smaller. Will they disappear? We hope so, but science hasn't reached that point yet.

REFERENCES

1. Phibbs B, Holmes R, Lowe C. Transient myocardial ischemia: The significance of dyspnea. *Am J Med Sci*. 1968;256:210–218.
2. Stern S. Symptoms other than chest pain may be important in the diagnosis of "silent ischemia," or "the sounds of silence." *Circulation*: 2005;111:e435–e437.

CHAPTER 9

The Heart Valves

STICKING AND LEAKING VALVES

The valves you read about in Chapter 2 are made of thin flaps of living tissue: they can become diseased like any other tissue. The effect of disease on the valves will take one of two forms.

The word **stenosis** refers to an abnormal narrowing of any kind of passage or opening. Stenosis of a valve means that the valve can't swing open as widely as it should. Sometimes this happens because the valve flaps are stuck together by adhesions—that is, by scar tissue that forms after an inflammation (Fig. 9–1).

Sometimes the flaps turn into heavy, rigid masses of scar tissue that are so stiff they can't swing apart normally (Fig. 9–2A). In either case, the blood is forced through an abnormally small orifice, like a large river running through a narrow canyon. **Regurgitation**, of course, means "leaking." When a physician says that a valve regurgitates, he or she could just as well say it leaks, but that wouldn't sound nearly as impressive. Normal valve flaps meet tightly at the edges, like perfectly milled doors. The blood can't go back into the chamber it came out of, so it has to move forward.

Imagine that a vandal went down the meeting edges of our two perfectly milled doors with a rasp file and a saw, cutting gouges and holes, so that when the door swung shut the wind whistled back through. That's exactly what disease processes can do to the edges of the valves. They can be scarred and gouged out of shape, so that when they swing shut there are holes and gaps that let the blood leak back into the chamber it just came out of (Fig. 9–2B). It's better to consider this subject one valve at a time.

Aortic Stenosis

This is the most dangerous of all valve lesions: it often leads to sudden death. Stenosis of the aortic valve was formerly caused by the scarring that follows rheumatic fever. This disease is now rare in the Western world and the great majority of cases of aortic stenosis at this time are the result of chalky degeneration, or sclerosis, of the aortic valve. The valve flaps become heavy and rigid and the valve opening may be no more

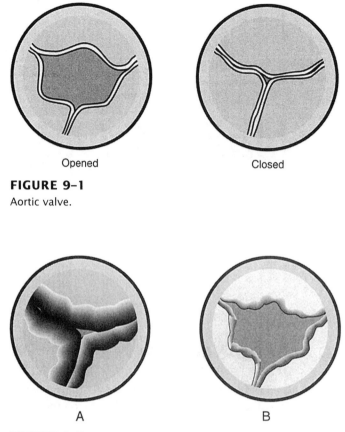

FIGURE 9-1
Aortic valve.

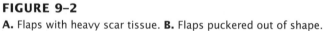

FIGURE 9-2
A. Flaps with heavy scar tissue. **B.** Flaps puckered out of shape.

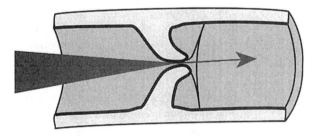

FIGURE 9-3
Aortic stenosis.

than a slit. This type of sclerotic, or rigid-degenerative, disease is almost always seen in older patients (Fig. 9–3).

When the heart has to force the entire blood supply of the body through a tiny opening, there are a number of consequences, all bad.

1. The blood supply to the brain is cut down. The patient will often become dizzy, or will actually faint, especially when exercising (Fig. 9–4).

2. The muscle of the left ventricle has to work against an enormous load. The muscle wall will enlarge for a time, but finally the pumping action of the ventricle will fail. Congestive heart failure follows swiftly (see Fig. 7–5 in Chap. 7).

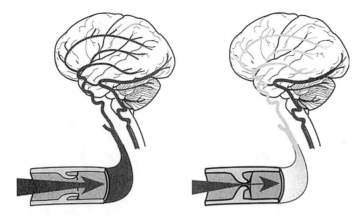

FIGURE 9-4
Reduced blood supply to the brain.

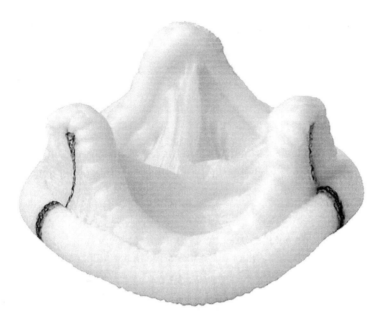

FIGURE 9-5
Bioprosthetic heart valve. These valves are constructed of porcine or bovine valvular tissue prepared with protective covering and mounted on a ring. This is a bioprosthesic heart valve. (Courtesy of St. Jude Medical)

3. The enormous muscle mass of the ventricle outruns its own coronary blood supply. The patient will begin to feel anginal pain.

When aortic stenosis begins to produce any of these symptoms, there is a 50% risk of sudden death within 2 years. Surgical replacement of the valve is urgent (Fig. 9–5). The results of surgery are very good, and the great majority of patients recover cardiac function to a large extent.

This excellent outcome arises from the fact that aortic stenosis puts a "pressure load" on the heart muscle, which hypertrophies, or thickens, in response. When the pressure load is removed, the heart muscle can revert to a normal state to a surprising degree.

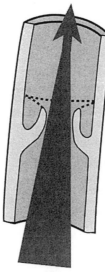

A normal amount
of blood is pumped out.

If the aortic valve leaks,
some of the blood flows
back into the left ventricle.

FIGURE 9–6
Aortic regurgitation.

Aortic Regurgitation

When the aortic valve leaks blood back into the left ventricle, the chamber has to work harder than normal. It has to pump the blood that leaked back out again together with the usual volume of blood it would have pumped anyway.

The seriousness of aortic regurgitation depends entirely on the volume of blood that leaks. If it's only one-half teaspoon (about 2 cc), for example, the patient can lead a normal life with a normal life expectancy. If it's a tablespoonful (16 cc), the heart will be overloaded. The patient will go into congestive heart failure and will die if the valve isn't replaced surgically (Fig. 9–6).

The only effect of aortic regurgitation is to overload the left ventricle and produce congestive heart failure. The only symptom of aortic regurgitation is shortness of breath.

Important warning about aortic regurgitation: **If a serious leak goes on too long, the ventricle is stretched past the point of no return**. Changes take place in the heart muscle so that it never regains normal function. Even after the valve is replaced surgically, some patients will die of progressive heart failure. This is because there has been a volume load imposed on the left ventricle by the mass of blood leaking back through the valve and the muscle is actually stretched in a way that damages the cells so that they never recover. Timing of valve replacement in aortic regurgitation is one of the most difficult decisions in cardiology. Measurement of the size of the left ventricle by echocardiography is one of the most important tests in helping the cardiologist make this decision.

Mitral Stenosis

This is always caused by the scarring of rheumatic fever. Since rheumatic fever is rare in the Western world, this valve lesion is becoming uncommon, but it still turns up as the result of rheumatic fever in earlier life. The edges of the valve flaps are stuck together with adhesions, so that the valve opening is sometimes no bigger than a ball-point pen. When this happens, the blood backs up into the lungs and the changes of

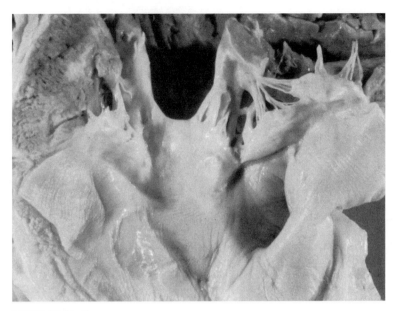

FIGURE 9–7
Rheumatic heart disease affecting the mitral valve. The two flaps of the mitral valve occupy the right-hand two thirds of the picture: they are thickened and white as a result of scarring and subsequent calcification. (Courtesy of Dr. Richard E. Sobonya, Pathology Department, University of Arizona Medical Center.)

congestive heart failure follow. In the later stages, the valve flaps may become heavy with scar tissue, so that they have the consistency of chalk or wood (Fig. 9–7).

The only treatment of mitral stenosis is surgical opening of the valve. It is very successful. In recent years the technique of balloon valvuloplasty has given excellent results. A catheter with two heavy balloons is threaded across the valve, the balloons are inflated, and the valve is literally torn open. This sounds brutal, but it works remarkably well. For many patients, balloon valvuloplasty is the best method. For others, valvuloplasty, or reconstruction of the diseased valve, is possible. If the valve is totally calcified into a hard chalky mass, it must be removed and an artificial valve implanted (see Fig. 9–5).

Mitral Regurgitation

Experience is teaching everyone that surgery for mitral regurgitation should be employed earlier than in the past. Just as with aortic regurgitation, the heart muscle is actually "stretched"—that is, overloaded—with an excess volume of blood. We now know that this kind of load produces irreversible changes in the heart muscle. Further, when the mitral valve is leaking, the ventricle has been pumping a significant volume of blood into the low-pressure system of the left atrium.

That doesn't involve much work. When the valve is repaired, however, this damaged ventricle has to pump blood against the much higher pressure of the aorta, and the weakened muscle simply can't handle the load.

The first thing that happens when blood leaks back through the mitral valve is that the left atrium enlarges, because it is forced to hold an abnormally large volume of blood. Since the pulmonary veins are wide open, with no valves, this increased blood volume is forced into the lungs with the usual results—congestive heart failure begins and the patient is short of breath (Fig. 9–8).

If the leak in the mitral valve is small, the patient can tolerate it throughout a normal life span. If it is large, the valve must be replaced surgically. Medical measures can

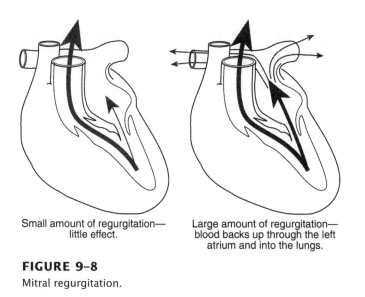

Small amount of regurgitation—
little effect.

Large amount of regurgitation—
blood backs up through the left
atrium and into the lungs.

FIGURE 9–8
Mitral regurgitation.

help to balance the effect of a large regurgitation for a time, but surgery will always be necessary for any significant mitral regurgitation.

Pulmonic Stenosis

Stenosis of the pulmonic valve is a rare, congenital phenomenon that often requires surgery (see Chap. 13). The same is true of tricuspid stenosis.

Tricuspid Regurgitation

With severe congestive heart failure, the backup of blood in the lungs causes a rise in pressure in the pulmonary artery and right ventricle. When the pressure in the right ventricle is high enough, the tricuspid valve, which is structurally weak, will leak back into the right atrium. This increased pressure will in turn back up throughout the veins (Fig. 9–9) and will force water out into the tissues. Thus, the result of tricuspid regurgitation will be the typical edema of right heart failure. Tricuspid regurgitation is almost always a secondary result of left heart failure. Left heart failure causes a rise in pressure in the vessels in the lungs, and this pressure is transmitted back through the pulmonary artery to the right ventricle. Tricuspid regurgitation due to actual disease of the valve is very rare.

INFECTIOUS HEART DISEASE

Any collection of living cells can be attacked by bacteria or viruses—the cells that make up the heart are no exception.

An infection will usually pick out one layer of the heart; for example, it may attack the pericardium, the myocardium, or the endocardium. (Rarely, all three may be involved.)

Pericarditis

Remember that the pericardium is the loose sac of tissue that holds the heart. Normally, it's a smooth, shiny membrane about 2 mm thick.

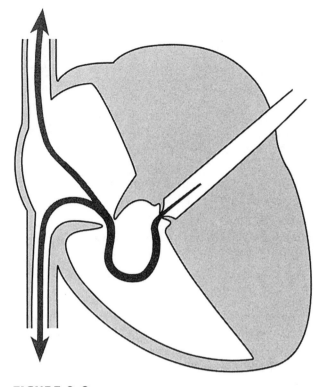

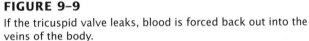

FIGURE 9–9
If the tricuspid valve leaks, blood is forced back out into the
veins of the body.

Any of the ordinary bacteria or viruses that produce sore throats, colds, pneumonia, or meningitis may attack the pericardium. To picture pericarditis, think of the way your throat looks when you have a bad sore throat. The surface of the pericardium will be red and raw and sometimes bloody, and fluid will ooze into the pericardial space, just the way fluid runs out of your nose when you have a cold. This fluid may be thin and clear, or bloody, or it may contain pus.

Pericarditis will usually cause pain as the heart moves against the raw, infected surface. This pain will be made worse by breathing, since the infected pericardium also rubs against the surface of the lungs.

How serious is pericarditis? It may be so mild that the patient thinks it's a bad cold with a "little ache in the chest." On the other hand, it may be very severe with sepsis and high fever. It all depends on what kind of germ attacks the pericardium.

At this time, most pericarditis is caused by viruses, and it's usually mild. In severe cases it may be necessary to insert a needle through the chest wall to identify the organism that's causing the infection. If a bacterium is present, antibiotics may halt the infection; if the disease is caused by a virus, there's no specific treatment except for rest and general support.

Very rarely, large amounts of fluid can form within the pericardium, pressing on the heart so that it can't pump normally (Fig. 9–10). In these cases, it is necessary to drain the fluid from the pericardial sac to relieve this pressure.

When tuberculosis was common, tuberculous pericarditis often left such heavy scars that the pericardium was plastered onto the heart, constricting it so that it couldn't function adequately. Surgery was necessary to remove the scars and free up the heart. Fortunately, the phenomenon of constrictive pericarditis is rare at this time.

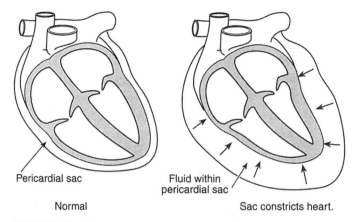

Pericardial sac

Normal

Fluid within
pericardial sac

Sac constricts heart.

FIGURE 9–10
When blood or fluid piles up in the pericardial sac, it can
constrict the heart dangerously. This is called tamponade.

Myocarditis

Inflammation of the myocardium is probably very common, but in mild cases it's hard
to be sure that it has happened. Any of the viruses lumped under the heading of "flu"
or "colds" can attack the heart muscle. When you've had an attack of flu that left you
tired and breathless for several weeks afterward, with an unusually rapid pulse when
you exercised, the chances are that the virus infected the heart muscle and left it
inflamed and temporarily weakened.

Most of the common infectious agents can and do attack the heart—muscle fungi,
one-celled creatures called trypanosomes, the spirochete of syphilis, the virus of glandu-
lar fever, the diphtheria germ, to name a few—but in the Western world today, it's safe to
say that over 90% of all cases of myocarditis are caused by viruses. Here's what happens.

A virus attacks the cells of the heart muscle. In the battle between virus and cell,
the muscle cells themselves change their chemistry just as if a soldier changed to an
enemy's uniform during a battle (Fig. 9–11).

As a result, the body's own defense cells now identify the heart muscle cells as
"enemy," treating the heart muscle cells as if they were foreign cells that didn't belong
there. The defense cells of the body (the lymphocytes) attack the heart muscle cells
and attempt to destroy them. Some heart muscle cells are indeed destroyed and others are damaged (Fig. 9–12).

There are no specific signs or symptoms. The patient will simply feel the effects of
a weakened ventricle: shortness of breath and general fatigue. The disease may be so

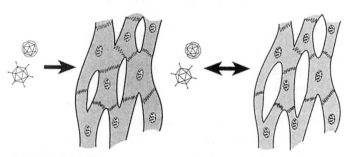

FIGURE 9–11
A virus attacks the heart muscle cells. In reaction to the virus,
the heart muscle cells may change their chemical character, like
soldiers putting on the wrong uniform.

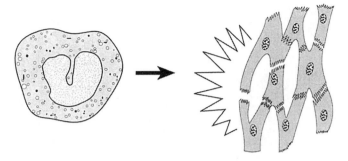

FIGURE 9–12
Lymphocytes attack heart muscle cells; some are destroyed,
some damaged.

mild that the patient is only aware of fatigue and rapid pounding of the heart for a few weeks. On the other hand, it can be fatal.

The diagnosis of myocarditis is made by ruling out other causes of impaired ventricular performance. A patient presents with heart failure: the valves and blood pressure are normal and the coronary arteries are wide open, but every test shows that the ventricle is weakened. The cardiologist will probably assume that myocarditis is the cause. In rare cases it is necessary to take a biopsy of the heart muscle through a catheter, but most of the time routine testing is enough.

Treatment

There is no specific treatment for viral myocarditis. The heart should be supported by drugs and by prolonged rest—sometimes for months. With this kind of intensive, prolonged management, many patients make gratifying recoveries. However, it's crucial to remember that there is no specific cure for the disease and that healing takes time.

Endocarditis

The endocardium is a smooth, shiny membrane, exactly like the lining of your mouth. When infection attacks this membrane, a specific and dangerous disease called endocarditis results. It's very common for bacteria to circulate in the bloodstream. They're released anytime tissues are hurt or roughly handled. Even brushing your teeth hard lets the bacteria from the mouth invade the blood and circulate for a time.

If there's a rough spot anywhere on the endocardium, bacteria can lodge there and begin to grow. The scars on a heart valve are a favorite nesting place. The bacteria form clotted blood around the scars, creating a kind of toxic nest. These masses of clotted blood and bacteria are called **vegetations**. They look very much like fungi growing on a tree.

The danger is that these vegetations are very fragile—sooner or later, pieces break off and circulate out through the arteries. They may land in the brain, the kidneys, the fingers, the toes, the spleen, and so on. These floating clots are little time bombs: they're loaded with bacteria and they form abscesses wherever they lodge. If the clots are large, they block off the blood supply and cause an infarct (Fig. 9–13). (Infarct is the death of tissue because the blood supply is cut off.)

Before the discovery of penicillin, nobody in the history of the human race ever recovered from endocarditis. It was always fatal—a more dangerous disease than cancer. Even with antibiotics it's still a dangerous disease, but now the mortality is under 30% for all cases.

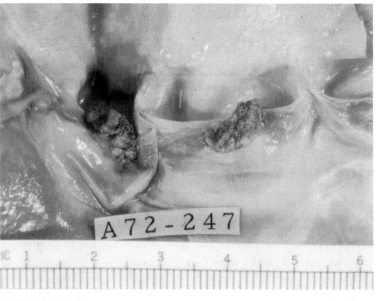

FIGURE 9–13
Vegetations of bacterial endocarditis growing on the leaflets of the aortic valve. The vegetations are dark, irregular masses growing on the smooth lining tissue of the valve. (Courtesy of Dr. Richard E. Sobonya, Pathology Department, University of Arizona Medical Center.)

There are two general clinical forms of the disease: acute and subacute endocarditis. Acute endocarditis is a swift, shattering infection, with rapid discharge of emboli and high fever. It is often caused by the staphylococcus. It can be cured, but treatment must be prompt and adequate. The danger of septic shock or fatal embolism is very high. Subacute endocarditis is still (despite some argument about terminology) a good descriptive classification. This form of the disease comes on gradually, over weeks or months. Low-grade fever and evidence of small clots in the blood vessels of the fingers, the kidneys, or other organs will be the clues that will alert the physician. Although this form of the disease would ultimately be fatal if not treated, there is more time to establish a diagnosis and organize an antibiotic program.

Who is at risk for endocarditis? First, anybody with an abnormality that affects the lining of the heart is at risk, such as

1. stenosis or regurgitation of the valves (especially regurgitation)
2. certain congenital heart lesions (see Chap. 13)
3. foreign bodies in the heart—artificial valves or pacemaker wires

Second, individuals who inject foreign substances into their veins risk developing endocarditis. Before the current drug epidemic swept the land, endocarditis occurred only in people with some abnormality of the lining of the heart. If the heart was structurally normal, bacteria circulating in the blood simply swept on past because they had no place to lodge. When anyone is idiotic enough to inject bacteria-laden chemicals into the blood through a dirty needle, endocarditis is likely to follow even though the heart is normal. The moral is obvious.

Treatment of endocarditis is based on prolonged use of the appropriate antibiotic— usually an 8-week course. "Appropriate antibiotic" means that the bacteria causing the infection have been detected in the blood and identified precisely. This often requires repeated blood sampling for culture of the bacterial growth in the laboratory. Physician and patient may need a great deal of patience, but the stakes are nothing less than life and death.

Prevention of Endocarditis

Prevention is everything! *Any* kind of injury or irritation to any body cavity will release bacteria into the bloodstream. "Any body cavity" means the mouth, the vagina, and the rectum. *Any* examination or surgical procedure of these areas must be considered to release bacteria into the bloodstream. If a patient has any of these risk factors, prophylactic antibiotics must be given on the morning of the day of the procedure and continued for 3 days thereafter.

What antibiotics? The antibiotic depends on the cavity: there are different kinds of germs in each. The physician must select an antibiotic appropriate to the area being treated and administer adequate amounts.

A patient who has any of the risk factors for endocarditis should be carefully instructed to remind all physicians of the need for endocarditis prophylaxis.

Special Note: Any dental procedure, including cleaning of the teeth, requires prophylaxis. Childbirth may result in massive invasion of bacteria from the vagina to the bloodstream. Endocarditis prophylaxis was formerly recommended in all cases of childbirth. Some recent studies have indicated this danger may be so small in modern settings that prophylaxis is indicated only if there is a specific source of infection.

Except for narcotic-related infections, endocarditis has been declining as a cause of death and illness throughout the Western world. Prevention and adequate treatment have shrunk this killer to about 10% of its former dimensions. It's not gone, but it's manageable.

MITRAL VALVE PROLAPSE

Until 1963, all of us who listened to hearts were baffled by some odd noises we heard. In the middle of systole, there might be odd clicking sounds, and sometimes late in systole we heard a murmur that sounded like someone giving a rising whoop from far away.

A South African cardiologist named John B. Barlow actually recorded these sounds from inside the heart with a microphone on the end of a catheter. He discovered that they were caused by a weakened mitral valve. It's the function of the mitral valve to hold tight against the pressure in the ventricle during systole so that no blood leaks back into the left atrium. The tissues holding the valve in place may be weak, or the valve leaflet itself may be too large, so that it's loose and "floppy." At the peak of systolic pressure, a weakened mitral valve may "let go" and pop back into the atrium a little. This is called prolapse (Fig. 9–14).

When the mitral valve prolapses, the physician may be able to hear a clicking noise. Naturally this will occur at or just after the peak of systolic pressure. If the prolapse is larger, there may be a murmur as a little blood leaks back into the atrium.

In the vast majority of cases, mitral valve prolapse doesn't mean a thing. In about 98% of cases, it isn't a significant form of heart disease because it doesn't cause symptoms and it isn't dangerous. As many as 20% of first-year female college students have been shown to have the click of mitral prolapse. They didn't need any medical care or further diagnostic study.

Severe mitral valve prolapse is rare. Sometimes a valve or its attachments can be so severely diseased that a great deal of blood leaks back into the left atrium. This is treated like any mitral regurgitation: with surgery.

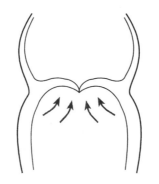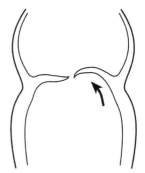

During systole the mitral valve has   Weakened mitral valve may give
to hold tight against the rising   way, or prolapse, up into the atrium.
pressure in the ventricle.

FIGURE 9–14
Mitral valve prolapse.

Severe mitral valve prolapse may be associated with chest pain that can be confused with the pain of coronary artery disease. Nobody is sure what causes this discomfort and some doubt that it exists. The pain is a nuisance, but that's all. It doesn't mean that anything's going to happen. It's the kind of pain you can treat with aspirin. Patients with severe mitral prolapse may also have abnormal rapid heart rhythms at times. These usually arise in the atria or the AV node, and are of the type called paroxysmal supraventricular tachycardia (see Chap. 12). Also, there's a rare form of prolapse that tends to run in families: in these patients, exercise may bring on ventricular tachycardia in short runs. These are the complications that come in rare, severe cases of mitral valve prolapse.

I heavily emphasize the harmless nature of most mitral valve prolapse for a reason. I've seen large numbers of patients frightened into invalidism because some physician heard a prolapse click. These unfortunate people were informed they had significant heart disease and were stuffed with strong cardiac medications. Some of them even underwent cardiac catheterization for no comprehensible reason. All too often the cardiac drugs made them sick and the fear of heart disease constricted their lives. All they really needed was reassurance, sometimes in large doses.

There is no question that mitral prolapse presents a risk for endocarditis. There is considerable question, however, about which type of prolapse presents a risk and how such patients can be identified. It is universally agreed that the risk is high in the severe type of prolapse, characterized by the typical "prolapse murmur"—the late systolic murmur characteristic of this particular abnormality. Prophylaxis should always be administered in such cases. When there is only a midsystolic click, the risk is probably lower, but the problem isn't simple. Some patients will have a click one day, a click plus murmur the next day, and simply a murmur on yet another day. This brings us to an editorial comment on endocarditis prophylaxis.

Endocarditis prophylaxis is simple, safe, and cheap. Modern prophylaxis consists of a few tablets of an antibiotic. Nit-picking arguments about the percentage of risk in a given setting are therefore foolish and possibly dangerous. If there is the slightest possibility of endocarditis, give prophylaxis! The consequences of not administering prophylaxis may be lethal. The logic is overwhelming: Use prophylaxis liberally!

CHAPTER **10**

The Autonomic or Automatic Nervous System

NERVES YOU DO NOT HAVE TO THINK ABOUT

In Chapter 7 on hypertension, the sympathetic nerves are described. These nerves are part of a larger system called the autonomic nervous system. It's time to describe it.

When you look at the light, the pupil of your eye gets smaller. You don't have to think about it—it just happens. The same thing happens when you bite a pickle and saliva forms, or when your stomach contracts to propel food along, or when your heartbeat speeds or slows. There are a multitude of functions your body takes care of automatically, through a special set of nerves called the autonomic (automatic) nervous system. There are two parts to this system: the sympathetic and parasympathetic nerves.

Sympathetic Nerves

The sympathetic nerves actually manufacture adrenaline and other chemicals like adrenaline at the nerve endings. When they are stimulated, you get exactly the effect you'd expect from a shot of adrenaline. The heart muscle contracts with more power, the heart beats faster, and the blood pressure rises.

Parasympathetic Nerves

The parasympathetic nervous system consists of one great nerve called the **vagus nerve**. The nerve endings of the vagus nerve release a chemical called acetylcholine. Generally, the effect of the vagus nerve is to slow things down. It's roughly opposite to the effect of the sympathetic nerves. To understand the effect of various diseases, drugs, and maneuvers on the heart, it's essential to understand how the sympathetic and vagus nerves affect heart function.

It's possible to stimulate the vagus nerve artificially. A small bundle of nerve tissue lies on each side of the neck, just under the jaw, in the fork of the carotid artery. It is called the carotid sinus.

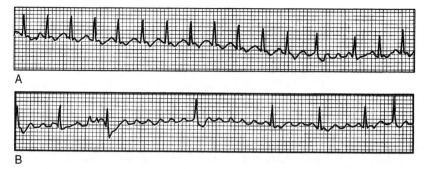

In strip A there is a rapid regular heartbeat with a rate of 125 bpm. From the first part of the strip, it would be very difficult to be sure that this wasn't a simple sinus tachycardia with one P wave for each QRS. Vagal stimulation produces block in the AV node so that no atrial impulses reach the ventricles for a long time. It is now clear that the atria are fluttering at a rate of 250 bpm. Note the long spaces between the third, fourth, and fifth QRS complexes in strip B. Even though the atrial impulses are bombarding the AV node very rapidly, they are blocked from reaching the ventricles for slightly over 2 seconds between these pairs of beats.

FIGURE 10–1
Effect of vagal stimulation on the AV node.

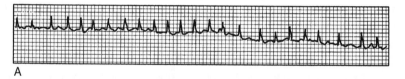

Note the rapid, irregular rhythm. This is atrial fibrillation: the atria are firing rapidly and irregularly, rather like a pinwheel on the Fourth of July. Electric impulses are bombarding the AV node about 425 times a minute—much too fast for each one to be conducted. Those that do make it through to the ventricles come in a wildly irregular rhythm with a rate that is often over 180 bpm. The heart cannot fill and empty efficiently with these shallow, rapid beats, and the patient usually goes into congestive heart failure.

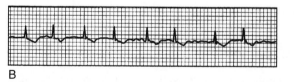

The ventricular rate has slowed to about 80 bpm and the patient is out of trouble. The atria are still fibrillating, but digitalis has stimulated the vagus nerve and this has produced a degree of block in the AV node. As a result, only a reasonable number of impulses reach the ventricles, the rate drops to normal, and the heart can pump efficiently.

FIGURE 10–2
Stimulation of the vagus by digitalis.

By pressing on this structure or by massaging it lightly, it is possible to stimulate the vagus nerve fibers that supply the heart. The sinus node may slow dramatically; conduction through the AV node may be depressed. (Either or both may happen.) This maneuver is often useful in the treatment of rapid heart action arising in the AV nodal tissue, since it turns off the rapid reciprocating circuit in the AV node that causes the rapid heartbeat. It is also helpful in diagnosing some arrhythmias (Fig. 10–1).

Certain drugs—for example, digitalis—exert much of their effect by stimulating the vagus nerve so that conduction through the AV node is depressed. From this point on in the book, the term **vagal effect** will be used often. It refers to the slowing of the sinus rate or depression of AV nodal conduction from overactivity of the vagus nerve (Fig. 10–2).

CHAPTER 11

The Electrocardiogram

INTERPRETATION OF THE ELECTROCARDIOGRAM

In Chapter 8 on coronary artery disease, the electrocardiogram (ECG) bowed on stage because it is very useful in diagnosing myocardial infarction and other complications of coronary artery disease. From this point on the ECG will appear frequently. It's time to become familiar with it.

When someone is lying quietly, the only muscle moving vigorously is the heart muscle. In Chapter 6, it was made clear that the heart muscle contracts because it has its own built-in electric circuit driving it. It's easy to record this electric circuit by placing electrodes on the surface of the body and attaching them to a suitable recording device (Fig. 11–1). If you wanted to take a complete picture of a building, you would have to walk around it with your camera, taking shots of the front, sides, and back. To take a complete picture of the electric field of the heart, you have to record 12 different views. This is done by recording from different pairs of electrodes at various points on the limbs and the chest (Fig. 11–2).

The passage of the activating wave across the tissues of the heart is recorded in sequence from top to bottom, or, more accurately, from the sinoatrial node across the atria, down the AV node, and through the ventricles.

START WITH THE SINOATRIAL NODE

The sinoatrial node fires and the electric wave starts across the atria. This produces the first wave of the ECG, called the P wave. The width of the P wave measures the time required for the wave to travel across the atria. Each small square on the ECG paper equals 0.04 second, so taking that measurement is easy (Fig. 11–3).

The wave next moves down the AV node. Nothing shows on the surface ECG during this period: there's a flat segment (Fig. 11–4).

After passing through the AV node, the wave enters the bundle branch system and darts across the ventricles very quickly, at about 4 meters per second. This produces the sharp up-and-down waves of the ventricular complex—the QRS complex (Fig. 11–5).

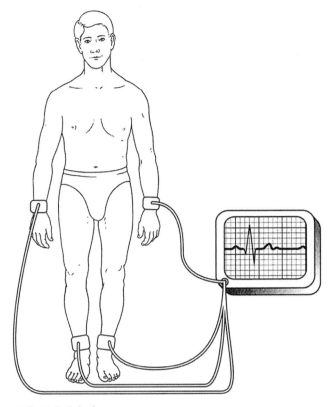

FIGURE 11–1
Placement of electrodes on the skin for recording the electric field of the heart.

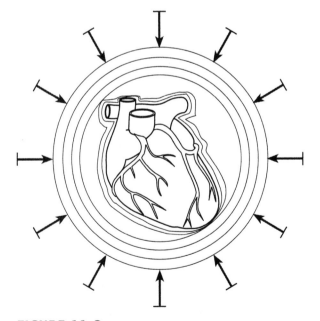

FIGURE 11–2
Twelve electrodes are placed on the chest and limbs.

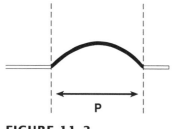

FIGURE 11–3
P wave.

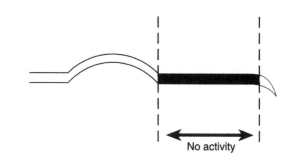

FIGURE 11–4
AV node.

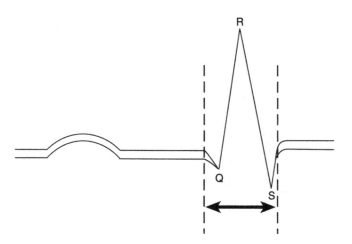

FIGURE 11–5
Width of QRS in a normal heart.

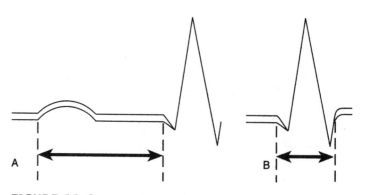

FIGURE 11–6
A. The PR interval. Normal is 0.12 to 0.20 second. B. QRS width.
Normal is 0.10 second or less.

Now, it's possible to measure three important intervals (Fig. 11-6):

1. The **PR interval**—the time from the beginning of the P wave to the end of the
   passage through the AV node.
2. The **QRS width**—the time it takes the electric impulse to travel across the
   ventricles.
3. The **QT interval**—the interval between the first deflection of the ventricular
   complex and the end of the T wave. (Sometimes there's no Q, so you just measure

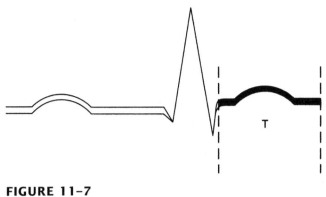

FIGURE 11-7
T wave.

from the first upstroke of the R.) This interval is very important: prolongation of the QT interval may indicate a potentially lethal abnormality.

There's a short pause after the wave reaches the end of its course, and then a return wave rolls back, restoring the conducting cells to normal. This is called the T wave (Fig. 11-7).

WAVE NAMES

If the first part of the ventricular complex is a down wave, it's called a Q wave. Any upward wave is called an R wave. Any downward wave after an R wave is called an S wave. Depending on the lead being recorded, it's possible to see any combination of these waves in a normal heart (Fig. 11-8).

The interval between the end of the QRS complex and the T wave is called the ST segment. It should be flat, exactly on the zero line, because there shouldn't be any electric activity during this period (Figs. 11-9 and 11-10).

Since the electric activation of the heart can be recorded with an accuracy to a hundredth of a second, the ECG can detect any abnormality of heart rhythm. It can also record failure of conduction through the various parts of the electric system. It should be possible to diagnose abnormalities of heart rhythm and conduction with almost 100% accuracy by means of the ECG. This is the first and most important use of the instrument.

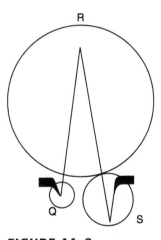

FIGURE 11-8
Nomenclature of Q, R, and S waves.

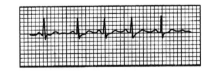

FIGURE 11-10
Normal ECG. Note that the segment between the end of the QRS and the beginning of the T wave is exactly at the baseline, that is, at the same level as the segment between the T wave and the P wave. To use medical jargon, "the ST segment is isoelectric."

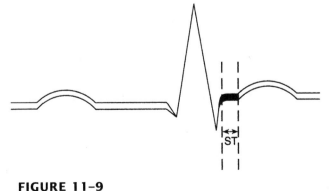

FIGURE 11-9
ST segment.

THE ECG AND MYOCARDIAL INFARCTION

Detecting myocardial infarction is the next most important function of the electrocardiogram. When the blood supply to the heart muscle is cut off, changes are recorded in the ECG almost at once.

When tissue loses its blood supply, it's injured. This injured tissue gives off a steady, small electric current called a current of injury. The only time this current can register during the heart cycle is during the quiet period—the ST segment. The current may cause either ST elevation or ST depression, depending on which lead you're looking at and where the injury is (Fig. 11–11).

As the heart muscle begins to die, the waves of the QRS complex will start to be affected. The most common change will be the appearance of a wide Q wave (one square or 0.04 second wide). The other waves of the complex may also be affected (Figs. 11–12 and 11–13).

Over the next 12 to 24 hours or more, all the injured tissue will either die or recover and the current of injury will disappear. The ST segments will come back to the zero line and the T wave will turn upside down, moving opposite to the way the ST segment went. This whole evolution may take as long as 2 weeks (Figs. 11–14 and 11–15).

This is the full-blown pattern of myocardial infarction. It would be handy if it appeared in all cases, but it doesn't. In possibly two thirds of all infarcts, these typical

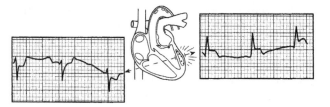

FIGURE 11–11

When heart muscle is infarcted, the ECG lead facing the infarct will show a rise in the ST segment because of a steady current of injury from the infarcted tissue. On the opposite side of the heart, this current of injury will register in an upside-down mirror image. Instead of being elevated it will be depressed. It's the same current, seen from the other side of the heart.

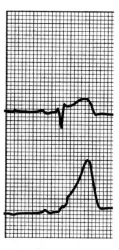

FIGURE 11–12

Earliest stage of myocardial infarction. Note the bizarre rise in ST segment in the leads facing the infarct. This is called hyperacute ST change.

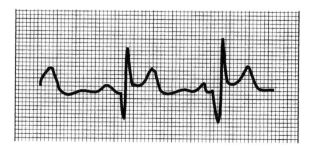

FIGURE 11–13

As the myocardial cells die, an initial negative deflection, or Q wave, appears. It is wide (more than 0.04 second). The ST segment is still elevated.

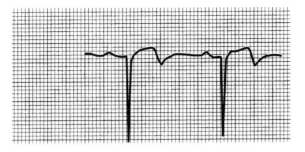

FIGURE 11–14
Final stage of evolution of myocardial infarct. There is
a Q wave, the ST segment has almost come back to
baseline, and the T wave is inverted.

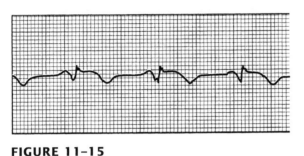

FIGURE 11–15
Another example of the end stage of evolution of a
myocardial infarct. Note the wide Q waves, the minimal
elevation of the ST segments, and the inverted
T waves.

changes are present. In most of the others, there is some progressive change, although
it's not the full-blown pattern. A T wave may invert, an ST segment may move up or
down, the QRS complex may change. The important thing is that there's progressive
change as the infarcted tissue dies. The clinician must combine these changes with the
symptoms and the blood enzymes to make a diagnosis.

Nonspecific Muscle Damage

Sometimes coronary artery disease, hypertension, or inflammation can leave
scarred heart muscle even though there hasn't been an infarct. This will often produce change in the shape of the T waves. In leads where the T waves should be
upright, they may invert or go to a plus–minus shape called "diphasic." The physician can state that there is some abnormality of the heart muscle, but he or she can't
say what kind (Fig. 11–16).

Chamber Enlargement

If the atria are large, the P wave will often be abnormally tall or wide (Fig. 11–17).

If a ventricle is enlarged (as, for example, in hypertension), the ECG lead over that
ventricle will record a tall R wave. There may also be a characteristic type of deformity
of the ST–T complex (Fig. 11–18).

Thus, enlargement of the various heart chambers can be recorded in the ECG,
although the accuracy isn't very high.

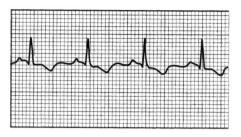

FIGURE 11–16
Nonspecific T wave change. Seeing an inverted T wave in certain leads, the electrocardiographer can say that there's been heart muscle damage. It's not possible to say what caused it or how extensive it is.

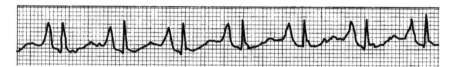

FIGURE 11–17
Atria enlargement. Tall P waves (more than 3 mm) with this "spiky" configuration are evidence of enlargement of the right atrium.

Pericarditis

Inflammation of the pericardium will almost always produce an injury current. This injury current comes from all around the surface of the heart, so that it will cause ST segment elevation in all leads. This is different from the changes in infarction, when the ST segments are up in some leads and down in others. There will be progressive change of the ST–T complex, very like the changes of infarction, except that the QRS is never involved.

Mineral Changes

Changes in the blood levels of potassium and calcium frequently produce changes in the ECG. Sometimes the ECG is more reliable than the blood level measurements in detecting dangerous changes in the cellular concentrations of these vital elements.

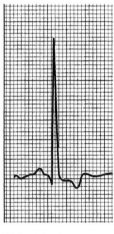

FIGURE 11–18
Ventricular enlargement. Tall R waves reflect a thickened ventricular myocardium. The ST–T deformity is of the type commonly seen with ventricular enlargement.

STRESS TESTING (EXERCISE TESTING)

When heart muscle isn't getting enough blood during an attack of angina pectoris it will often produce an injury current. This current will cause deflection of the ST segment of the ECG. It's possible to produce this situation artificially by driving the heart to a higher workload while observing the electrocardiogram. With the higher workload, the heart muscle will need more blood. If a coronary artery is diseased, the extra blood flow isn't available, and an injury current may appear on the ECG.

The simplest way to do this is to have the patient exercise on a treadmill or other exercise machine while the ECG is recorded continuously.

It's also important to record blood pressure at frequent intervals and to listen to the heart after exercise for abnormal sounds, or "gallops."

Exercise is continued until the ECG records an injury current or until the patient feels anginal pain. If there is no pain, and if the ECG remains normal, exercise is continued until the pulse rate reaches a maximal number calculated by age (Fig. 11–19).

Adequate exercise testing requires that a full 12-lead ECG be recorded during and after exercise. In the early days of stress testing, only 1 or 2 leads were recorded and much information was missed.

How accurate is stress testing? Everyone has heard stories about a patient who had a normal stress test only to suffer a heart attack a few weeks later. This is perfectly possible—the stress test isn't a crystal ball, and it can only record what has happened up to that point. In the best hands, stress testing is about 75% accurate—that is, if there is significant coronary artery disease, there is about a 75% chance that the stress test will detect it. There will be an error of at least 25%, including both "false positives" and "false negatives." In other words, even if a patient has a normal stress exercise test, there is still a chance that significant coronary artery disease is present.

On the other hand, an abnormal stress test doesn't necessarily mean coronary artery disease. There are many conditions that can produce a false-positive result. These conditions should be clearly understood by anyone involved in stress testing.

1. **Digitalis.** If a normal person takes digitalis and then exercises, there will be changes in the ST segment, just as if coronary artery disease were present. This is purely the result of the effect of the drug and has nothing to do with heart disease. Stress testing should never be performed on a patient taking digitalis. The drug should be discontinued for 2 weeks before stress testing.

2. **Preexcitation.** In the peculiar electrocardiographic syndrome known as preexcitation, abnormal tissues bypass the AV node. In these patients, stress testing is useless for detection of coronary artery disease since there usually will be abnormal ST deviation even when the coronary arteries are normal.

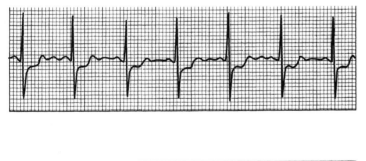

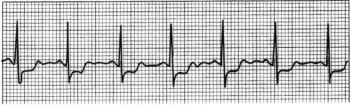

FIGURE 11–19
Two simultaneous leads recorded during stress testing. The ST segments are depressed 3 mm below the baseline. Sustained depression is also an important feature. This degree of ST change during stress testing is strong evidence that an area of heart muscle is not receiving enough blood for the increased workload, presumably as a result of coronary artery disease.

3. **Syndrome X.** Middle-aged females have a very high incidence of false-positive stress tests. This may be part of syndrome X, or pseudoangina (see Chap. 17).

This is only a partial list of conditions that interfere with stress testing; there are many others.

Scoring a Stress Test

If the ST segments move up or down 2 mm or more, the test is more likely to be accurate and the disease is more likely to be severe than if lesser deviations are recorded.

If pain or ST change appear at a low level of exercise, there is likely to be severe coronary artery disease.

Normally, the systolic blood pressure rises and falls with the pulse rate. If the systolic pressure falls with exercise, especially if ST change is also present, there is a high risk of disease of the left main coronary artery or of all three vessels.

Variations of Stress Testing

Some patients can't walk through a stress test because of disease of the lower extremities. Others can't exercise very much because of lung disease (for example, emphysema). Here are three methods that get around these problems.

Radioisotope Testing

The radioactive element thallium-201 will be picked up by healthy heart cells but not by cells that have an inadequate blood supply. This difference can be used to detect subnormal coronary blood flow. The patient is exercised to the point of pain, ST changes, or maximum pulse, and the isotope is injected. If some heart muscle fails to receive enough blood at that point, the isotope won't be picked up and a blank spot will show up when the heart is scanned. Another scan is performed 2 hours later when the blood supply should have returned to normal. If the blank spot has disappeared, it means that there was temporarily inadequate blood flow to an area of heart muscle—in other words, coronary artery disease. This method has not yielded the results that were hoped for, but it is sometimes helpful.

When thallium-201 scanning is combined with injection of the chemical dipyridamole, the results are about as good as with conventional treadmill testing. The advantage of the dipyridamole test is that the patient has to walk only 2 or 3 minutes. There are, however, some side effects to the injection of dipyridamole in a few patients, so the method must be used with caution.

Stress Echocardiography

Stress echocardiography combines a stress test with echocardiograms recorded before and immediately after testing, and has added greatly to the accuracy of the method. Abnormality of motion, loss or diminution of motion, systolic thinning of heart muscle (remember that heart muscle, like any muscle, ought to thicken when it contracts), or paradoxical motion of heart muscle all indicate acute lack of adequate blood supply. Stress echocardiography is as accurate as isotope study. In addition, it's much cheaper and easier to apply. If the patient can't walk on a treadmill, chemical stressing with dobutamine or dipyridamole can be used, just as in isotope testing.

Holter Monitor Recordings

The Holter monitor is Montana's contribution to modern cardiology. Eric Holter, an inventor in Helena, decided he'd like to know what his ECG looked like when he was exercising, or angry, or eating, or sleeping—not just when he was lying on his physician's examining table. He also realized how important it could be to record temporary disorders of rhythm or transient changes in the ST segment during angina. To do this, it was obviously necessary to record the ECG continuously for long periods of time—12 to 24 hours.

After years of work, the modern Holter monitor emerged as a valuable diagnostic tool that is used all over the world. Three electrodes are attached to the patient's chest and a small recording device is slung from a strap worn over one shoulder, much like a camera or a pair of binoculars. The ECG is recorded continuously on tape: this can be played back on a screen that permits continuous viewing. Any parts of interest can be recorded on regular ECG paper.

Early models of the Holter monitor were excellent for detecting disorders of rhythm and conduction. Later models employing two ECG leads have permitted accurate recording of ST segment changes of the type that occurs during angina.

The patient is provided with a diary so that symptoms can be recorded together with the time they appeared. Time intervals are also displayed on the Holter monitor, permitting precise correlation of symptoms with ECG change.

The Holter monitor records the heartbeat for a maximum of 24 hours, but many times a patient will describe an abnormal heartbeat that occurs only once or twice a week. This was a problem until the last few years, when a remarkable instrument called the event recorder was perfected. This is a small recording device about twice as big as an old-fashioned pocket watch. It's attached to the patient by two recording electrodes, just like the Holter monitor, but with one important difference: the event recorder starts recording when the patient pushes a button on the device. It goes back 5 minutes and records every heartbeat while the patient is actually feeling symptoms. This is a major breakthrough in the diagnosis of abnormalities of heart rhythm: it has made many older, more expensive, and sometimes dangerous techniques obsolete.

CHAPTER 12

Cardiac Arrhythmias

To understand the disorders of heart rhythm, it's essential to see them recorded in the electrocardiogram. Without this remarkable device, modern diagnosis and treatment of cardiac arrhythmias would be impossible.

NORMAL SINUS RHYTHMS

Logic will tell you what should appear in the ECG. Each impulse starts in the sinus node and travels across the atria, down the AV node, and through the ventricles, following the same track, moving at the same speed.

As a result, P waves will appear at regular intervals. Each P wave will be followed at identical intervals by QRS complexes and T waves. Every beat will look exactly like every other beat (Fig. 12–1).

SINUS ARRHYTHMIA

Take your pulse by putting two fingers on your wrist, just below the thumb. When you feel the pulse, take a deep breath in and let it out. The pulse will probably speed up as you inhale and slow as you exhale. This is a normal phenomenon, caused by reflexes

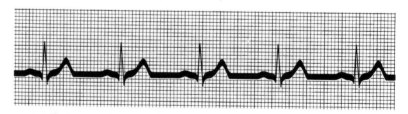

FIGURE 12–1
P waves appear at regular intervals. Each P wave is followed by a ventricular complex. The PR interval is about 0.15 second (normal). The width of the QRS is 0.08 second (normal). All criteria for normal sinus rhythm are met.

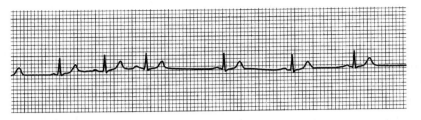

FIGURE 12–2

Sinus arrhythmia. All the beats are identical and the intervals are normal, but the space between beats varies as the heart speeds and slows with breathing. This is a normal phenomenon.

triggered by breathing. It can be quite pronounced, especially in young people. It should never be confused with a serious arrhythmia (Fig. 12–2).

ECTOPIC BEATS

The word *ectopic* means "outside the normal site." An ectopic pregnancy, for example, arises outside the uterus.

If the sinus node were the only pacemaker of the heart, higher life would have vanished from the earth a long time ago. The cells of the sinus node can become sick and may fail to fire, and if there were no other source of a heartbeat, life would end. Fortunately, there are hundreds of reserve pacemakers in the heart: tiny areas of tissue that can discharge a beat if needed. The heart is just like a car with 10 extra coils and 500 extra sparkplugs, organized in "fail-safe" systems. These ectopic pacemakers are scattered through the atria, the AV node, and the ventricles (Fig. 12–3).

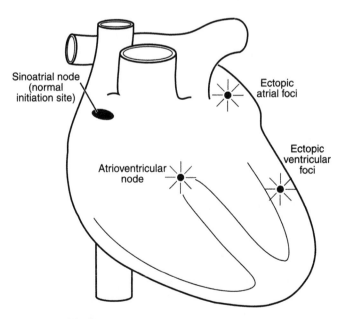

FIGURE 12–3

Beats can originate in four different places. It is usually simple to recognize the origin of beats. Clinically, it is important to differentiate between ventricular beats and those arising in the AV node or atria.

EXTRASYSTOLES

Everyone has them. You feel your heart "skip a beat"; there's an odd pause and you wonder if your heart is going to start again. What happens is that one of the ectopic pacemakers becomes "irritable" and fires early, when it isn't needed. The ectopic beat cuts into a normal sinus rhythm like this:

beat   beat   beat   beatBEAT   beat

The heart pauses after the early ectopic beat, and the next normal beat comes in where it would have if there had been a normal beat instead of the ectopic one—hence the pause (Fig. 12–4). It's easy to detect an ectopic beat on the ECG. It's also easy to tell exactly what part of the heart an ectopic beat comes from—that is, whether it comes from the atria, the AV node, or the ventricles. The pattern on the ECG is specific. Here are the rules:

1. If an ectopic beat arises in the top half of the heart, it will follow the normal track down across the ventricles. In other words, the ventricular track of an ectopic beat arising in the top half of the heart will look exactly like the ventricular track of a normal sinus beat. Like the sinus beat, it will be narrow—less than 0.12 second—because the ectopic impulse is conducted along the "fast track" in the ventricles at 4 meters per second. Beats arising in the top half of the heart are called **supraventricular beats** because they arise above the ventricles (Fig. 12–5). Figures 12–6 and 12–7 illustrate the phenomenon of atrial ectopic beats.

2. If an ectopic beat arises in the ventricles outside the normal conducting system, it has to move slowly because it's outside the normal track, like a car on a muddy detour. The impulse moves directly through the muscle of the left ventricle at 0.5 meter per second, or about one eighth of normal speed. Since the impulse takes a long time to move across the ventricles, the track on the ECG will be wide; it will always include at least three time lines or 0.12 second, never less. Because the activating wave is following a winding, complicated, backward track across the ventricles, the shape of the QRS and T waves will be completely different from the shape of normal beats (Fig. 12–8). Figure 12–9 illustrates the obvious differences in electrocardiographic pattern between supraventricular and ventricular ectopic beats.

It's often possible to tell whether ectopic beats arise in the atria or in the AV node, but that's not important at this point. What is important is to know that:

1. There are ectopic beats.
2. They arise in all parts of the heart.
3. Beats from the top of the heart are narrow and those from the bottom are wide.

It's also important to know that ectopic beats are a normal phenomenon. They feel strange, but they don't mean anything and they very rarely need treatment.

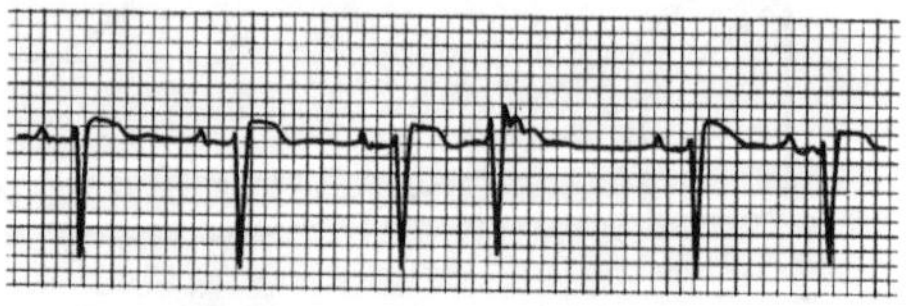

FIGURE 12–4
Normal sinus rhythm interrupted by an early beat (the fourth). This beat is caused by the premature discharge of an ectopic pacemaker.

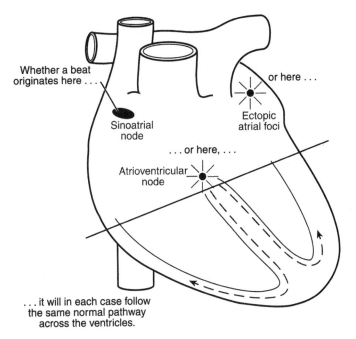

FIGURE 12–5

Supraventricular (atrial or nodal) beats. The ventricular complex will therefore be normal. It is not vital to distinguish between atrial beats and nodal beats. The important thing is to distinguish between beats arising above the bifurcation of the bundle of His and those arising somewhere in the ventricles.

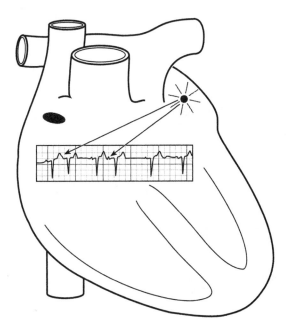

FIGURE 12–6

Premature atrial beats. The second and fourth beats arise from an ectopic focus in the atria. In each, there is a premature P wave followed by a normal QRS. The QRS is exactly like the QRS of the sinus beats because the activating impulse follows the normal track down the bundle branches and through the ventricles. Note that the premature, ectopic P waves have a different shape from the P waves of the sinus beats at the end of the strip.

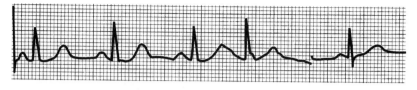

FIGURE 12-7

Normal sinus rhythm interrupted by a premature beat (the fourth). The QRS complex of the early beat looks like the QRS of the normal sinus beats. The early beat must come from the top half of the heart—the atria of the AV node. In this case, there's a tiny P wave hidden in the T wave just before the early beat; therefore, it must come from the atria.

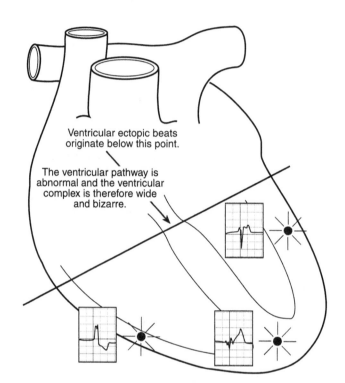

Ventricular ectopic beats originate below this point.

The ventricular pathway is abnormal and the ventricular complex is therefore wide and bizarre.

FIGURE 12-8

Ventricular beats. If the beat originates anywhere below the point indicated by the arrow, the ventricular complex will be abnormal in contour. The impulse must travel a "backward" or eccentric path through the ventricles. The complex inscribed by such an impulse will therefore be wide and bizarre in shape. There will be no P wave preceding the ventricular complex. The shape of the ectopic ventricular beat is determined by the point of origin within the ventricles. Each ectopic focus has its own characteristic pattern; three are depicted.

PAROXYSMAL TACHYCARDIA

Sometimes an ectopic focus goes on firing, rapidly and regularly, for a long time—minutes, hours, or even days. (A **paroxysm** is something that starts and stops abruptly. **Tachycardia** means a rapid heart rate.) The change is like this:

beat   beat   beat   beat   beatbeatbeatbeat

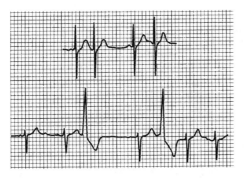

FIGURE 12–9

The top strip shows premature beats with a normal, narrow QRS complex appearing every other beat. These are supraventricular beats—they must arise in the atria or the AV node. The bottom strip shows premature beats arising in the ventricles. Note the characteristic wide, bizarre shape of the whole QRST complex compared to the shape of the normal sinus beats.

and so on for some time. The rate may be as high as 260 to 270 beats per minute (bpm) or as low as 130 to 140 bpm. This kind of beating is called paroxysmal tachycardia.

Like ectopic beats, paroxysmal tachycardia can arise from the atria, the AV node, or the ventricles (Fig. 12–10). The most important thing to know about a paroxysm of tachycardia is which part of the heart it arises in. If it arises in the top half of the heart, it isn't serious. Paroxysmal supraventricular tachycardia often appears in people with otherwise normal hearts, and it's easy to treat.

If paroxysmal tachycardia arises in the ventricles, it's always serious. Paroxysmal ventricular tachycardia almost always arises in damaged hearts, and it can threaten life. When it appears, a careful search should be made for some form of associated heart disease.

To make the distinction between the two types of paroxysmal tachycardia, you use the same trick you used in analyzing ectopic beats. If the ventricular complexes during a paroxysmal tachycardia are *narrow*, the tachycardia arises in the top half of the heart, and it's the harmless variety (Fig. 12–11). If the ventricular complexes are *wide*, the tachycardia almost certainly arises in the ventricles, and it's dangerous (Fig. 12–12). There are rare exceptions to this rule, but only a skilled electrocardiographer can make the distinction.

If you can count to three, you can tell the difference between supraventricular and ventricular tachycardia. The complexes of ventricular tachycardia will always be three squares wide (0.12 second); supraventricular tachycardia complexes will be less than three squares wide.

A patient will almost always feel some sensation when paroxysmal tachycardia starts—maybe a "pounding in the chest" or a "feeling as if the heart is running away." If the tachycardia is ventricular, the patient may become dizzy or start to lose consciousness. It's practically always possible to stop paroxysmal tachycardia with medicine, but there's a caution. The right treatment for supraventricular tachycardia may be very wrong for ventricular tachycardia and may even kill the patient.

The only way to tell the difference between the two varieties is to record an electrocardiogram while the tachycardia is going on. "Blind" treatment without a precise

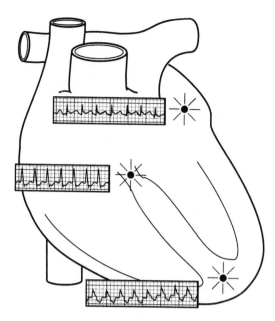

FIGURE 12–10

Paroxysmal tachycardia. When an ectopic pacemaker discharges rapidly and regularly, paroxysmal tachycardia is the result. Like premature beats, the tachycardias can originate in the atria, AV junction, or ventricles. The three types are differentiated by applying the same criteria one applies to premature beats. The rate may vary from 140 to 300 beats per minute.

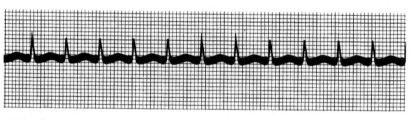

FIGURE 12–11

Paroxysmal tachycardia arising in the atria or the AV node. The rhythm is perfectly regular, the rate is 160, and the QRS complexes are narrow, meaning that they're following a normal track across the left ventricle.

diagnosis may be useless or dangerous. The moral is obvious: it's often possible to stop a paroxysmal tachycardia with medication. *Adenosine*, a drug that blocks the AV node for about 6 seconds, will almost always stop AV nodal reentrant tachycardia—which is the commonest type of supraventricular tachycardia. (Remember, the term *supraventricular* means "narrow beat tachycardia.")

Drugs used now for ventricular tachycardia include the very safe, old reliable *lidocaine* or the newer and very powerful *amiodarone*.

If paroxysmal supraventricular tachycardia recurs, drug therapy with digitalis, beta blockers, or calcium blockers is often effective. If drugs don't work, the patient should be sent to a good electrophysiology laboratory. (See the section later in this chapter called "Invasive Treatment of Arrhythmias.")

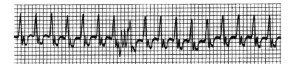

FIGURE 12–12
Paroxysmal tachycardia arising in the ventricles.
The beats look like ventricular ectopic beats, which,
of course, is what they are.

Amiodarone is the only drug used today to prevent recurrence of ventricular arrhythmias: older drugs such as procaine amide and quinidine have fallen into disuse because of rare but dangerous complications. In fact, even amiodarone must be used with careful supervision because of toxic side effects.

Again, recurrent ventricular arrhythmias that resist drug therapy can be treated by invasive methods, but the results aren't as good as with the supraventricular type.

Important Note: *Supraventricular tachycardias don't necessarily mean heart disease: they frequently occur in patients with otherwise normal hearts, and they never threaten life. Ventricular tachycardias of the common type almost always indicate heart disease and they indicate an urgent need for careful and thorough study.*

If medicine doesn't work, the tachycardia can be halted by a timed electric shock. Equipment to deliver this type of shock is available in every hospital and emergency room in the country and the technique is simple and safe.

ATRIAL FIBRILLATION

Imagine that you're looking at a beating heart. The atria are contracting regularly, in rhythm with the ventricles. Now imagine that the atria stop their regular beat and begin a fine, fast twitching motion. This kind of abnormal motion is called **fibrillation**. The electrocardiogram records fine, fast, irregular waves—just what you'd expect (Fig. 12–13).

The electric waves from the atria are hitting the AV node very rapidly and irregularly, like a shower of sparks from a pinwheel. They hit the AV node about 425 times a minute. The AV node cannot possibly conduct that fast. The cells in the AV node perform actual work with each passage. This work leaves them tired, and they can't conduct another impulse until they've had time to recover. This period is called the **refractory period**.

When fibrillating impulses are banging at the AV node 425 times a minute, many of these impulses will arrive when the cells are fatigued, or refractory from the previous passage, and the impulses won't be conducted. Only those impulses that find the AV node cells ready to conduct will reach the ventricles, and this is a matter of pure chance. The ventricular rhythm will therefore be completely irregular. "Like 'shave-and-a-haircut-six-bits' repeated fast a lot of times" was the way one of my interns put it. Good description. **Delirium cordis**, or "delirium of the heart," was the term physicians used a couple of hundred years ago to describe the fast, wildly irregular pulse (see Fig. 12–13).

Atrial fibrillation is dangerous because it drives the ventricles too fast. They can't pump efficiently. Imagine trying to squeeze water out of a bulb syringe. You could do pretty well squeezing 60 or 80 times a minute, but if you suddenly started twitching your hand a couple of hundred times a minute, you wouldn't pump much water. The syringe would never have a chance to fill between beats. This is what happens with atrial fibrillation: the pumping action of the heart fails, blood backs up into the lungs, and congestive heart failure follows (Fig. 12–14).

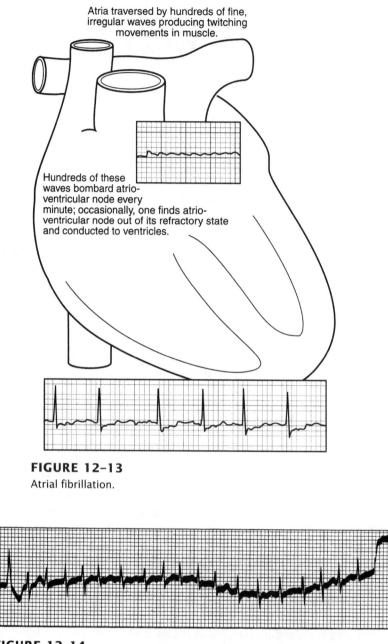

FIGURE 12–13
Atrial fibrillation.

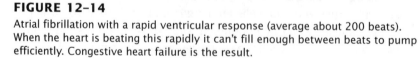

FIGURE 12–14
Atrial fibrillation with a rapid ventricular response (average about 200 beats).
When the heart is beating this rapidly it can't fill enough between beats to pump
efficiently. Congestive heart failure is the result.

The first step in treatment is to slow the heart rate by slowing conduction through
the AV node. This is done with digitalis, the oldest known cardiac drug. Digitalis actually
poisons the AV node so that it can't conduct too fast. By giving the right dose, it's possible to bring the ventricular rate down to normal and relieve the congestive heart failure.

Calcium-blocking drugs and beta-blocking drugs will also slow conduction through
the AV node and are often used today. Both these drugs, however, can drop blood pressure, and beta blockers can depress ventricular function, so digitalis is preferable in the
acute setting. For chronic control of rate with atrial fibrillation, it's essential to combine
digitalis with a calcium blocker or a beta blocker for one very practical reason: digitalis

will control the heart rate with atrial fibrillation when the patient is at rest but as soon as the patient begins to exercise, the digitalis effect is lost or diminished. This happens because exercise stimulates the sympathetic nervous system, whereas digitalis works by stimulating the opposing system (i.e., the parasympathetic nerves, chiefly the vagus).

There's a debate going on today about the proper management of chronic atrial fibrillation.

There are two potential approaches:

1. Convert the patient to a normal sinus rhythm and attempt to maintain that rhythm with medication.

2. Simply control the rate with medication and give anticoagulants to prevent discharge of blood clots.

Some simple rules apply.

First, if the atrial fibrillation comes on suddenly with an obvious cause (overactive thyroid gland, congestive heart failure) it's sensible to correct the cause and then try to restore a normal heart rhythm. Caution: If the atrial fibrillation has been going on more than 48 hours, anticoagulant therapy to suppress blood clots should be given for 3 weeks before any attempt is made to convert to a normal rhythm. If the atrial fibrillation has only been going on for a day or so, it's reasonable to try to convert the heart to a normal rhythm as quickly as possible. Conversion to sinus rhythm can be achieved by drugs (see below) or by electroshock. (Atrial fibrillation produced by heavy drinking or what the British call "Monday morning heart" is a prime example of a condition calling for prompt cardioversion.)

Second, if atrial fibrillation is chronic and no specific cause can be detected, the best course at this time appears to be to let the patient go on fibrillating, control the rate to keep it within normal bounds, and administer anticoagulant therapy.

A number of drugs are available to convert to sinus rhythm and maintain it, but they all carry a certain risk. Sotalol, mexiletine, procainamide, disopyramide, flecainide, quinidine, and amiodarone all present a risk of about 1% per year of potentially catastrophic arrhythmia (torsade).

As an interesting note about physicians and medical fads, quinidine is one of the oldest cardiac drugs we have and it's very effective early in atrial fibrillation. So is procainamide which is practically the same as quinidine in action and toxicity. These two drugs are much more effective in early cardioversion than the others listed. Amiodarone isn't very effective at all in cardioverting to a sinus rhythm, although it's useful in maintaining a sinus rhythm once it's been established. Physicians, however, are swayed by drug company advertisements and whatever is new tends to be in vogue, like fashions, so quinidine and procainamide have fallen into disuse. The British and other Europeans, however, are now "rediscovering" quinidine, so the fad cycle may be expected to swing that way again (Fig. 12–15).

Causes of Atrial Fibrillation

The competent physician will always look for a cause and treat it. Overactivity of the thyroid gland can cause atrial fibrillation; so can stretching of the atria when diseased valves cause back pressure. When hypertension causes heart failure, the pressure in the atria will rise and this, again, can lead to fibrillation. When there is a specific cause, of course, it should always be corrected. Sometimes there is no cause that can be discovered; atrial fibrillation can appear in a heart that seems otherwise normal.

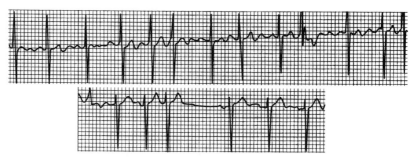

FIGURE 12–15
Conversion of atrial fibrillation to normal sinus rhythm as a result of drug therapy (quinidine). The top strip shows atrial fibrillation; on the right-hand side of the bottom strip, normal sinus rhythm has resumed.

Blood Clots and Atrial Fibrillation

Whenever blood stagnates, it tends to clog—very much like gelatin hardening. In fibrillating atria, the blood isn't being pumped cleanly and forcefully, and it tends to stagnate in the corners and recesses of the atria. Blood clots form. These clots are fragile: you could break them off by touching them. Pieces of these clots often do break off and float away in the bloodstream. They are dangerous—wherever clots lodge, they cut off the blood supply to the tissue downstream, and the tissue dies. If they lodge in the brain, clots cause a stroke. They can cause infarcts in the kidneys, the spleen, the adrenal glands, or, indeed, any organ of the body. Clots that lodge in the arms or legs can cause gangrene.

Anticoagulants, or drugs that keep blood from clotting, should be administered in practically all cases of atrial fibrillation. There's been a great deal of study on the subject of which patients should be given anticoagulants and everyone's now agreed on the guidelines.

First, when chronic atrial fibrillation is present, *any* patient with *any* kind of organic heart disease should be carried on Coumadin. "Heart disease" includes simple high blood pressure as well as coronary disease, valvular disease, diseases of heart muscle, and all forms of congenital disease except the type of atrial septal defect called ostium secundum (see Chap. 13).

Second, anyone with chronic atrial fibrillation over the age of 65 should be maintained on Coumadin. One large-scale study suggests that anyone over 60 should be maintained on the drug.

Third, if the fibrillation is caused by an overactive thyroid gland, the danger of a clot is extremely high. The patient should be started acutely on heparin, which works fast, and then maintained on Coumadin.

On the other hand, if the patient has what the British call "lone atrial fibrillation"—that is, atrial fibrillation in a patient under 65 with absolutely no evidence of heart or thyroid disease—anticoagulants are not necessary. Aspirin alone is all the protection these patients need.

ATRIAL FLUTTER

Atrial flutter is a "first cousin" to atrial fibrillation. Try opening and shutting one hand as fast as you can with a rapid, regular motion. This is what the atria do when they flutter. They stop their normal beat and go into a rapid "flapping" motion, like the wings of a bird. This motion is different from fibrillation because it's perfectly regular and it's slower—never more than 300 bpm in the adult heart.

The AV node can't conduct 300 times a minute, so only every other beat comes through to the ventricles. The resulting rate of 150 bpm is still too fast for good function, of course, and atrial flutter often causes congestive heart failure. It's not a rhythm patients are comfortable with; they always complain of "pounding" or "racing" of the heart (Fig. 12–16).

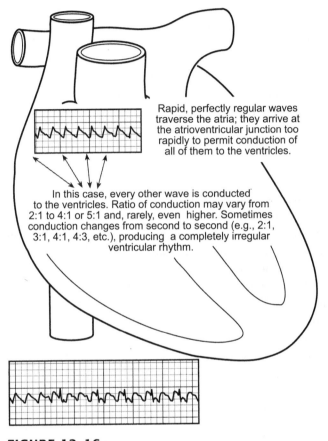

Rapid, perfectly regular waves traverse the atria; they arrive at the atrioventricular junction too rapidly to permit conduction of all of them to the ventricles.

In this case, every other wave is conducted to the ventricles. Ratio of conduction may vary from 2:1 to 4:1 or 5:1 and, rarely, even higher. Sometimes conduction changes from second to second (e.g., 2:1, 3:1, 4:1, 4:3, etc.), producing a completely irregular ventricular rhythm.

FIGURE 12–16
Atrial flutter with 2:1 conduction from the atria to the ventricles. The atrial rate is 300 bpm and the ventricular rate is 150—the most common pattern of atrial flutter.

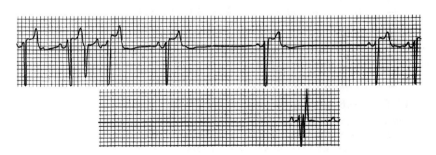

FIGURE 12–17
Sick sinus syndrome. The sinus rhythm suddenly slows. There are pauses between beats of 3 to 6 seconds.

Flutter is treated much like fibrillation. First, the heart rate is slowed by depressing the AV node so that it can't conduct very fast. Then the flutter is converted to a normal sinus rhythm by quinidine, procainamide, or electroshock. Fortunately, it's almost always possible to convert flutter to a normal sinus rhythm. The risk of clots with flutter is at least as high as with atrial fibrillation and the same measures should be taken to prevent them.

HEART BLOCK AND THE SICK SINUS SYNDROME

Everything so far has been about hearts going too fast. This section will be about hearts going too slow.

The sinus node is the normal pacemaker of the heart. It is made of cells that can sicken and die, like every other part of the body. When this happens, the sinus node may slow its rate so much that the heart doesn't pump an adequate amount of blood. The most common symptom of this kind of slowing will be dizziness or faintness since the brain isn't receiving enough oxygen. Sometimes the heart may slow abruptly and the patient may faint (Fig. 12–17).

Rarely, an abnormally slow heart rate may produce congestive heart failure or make it worse, and even more rarely, it can make angina worse, with relief when the rate returns to normal. Sometimes a very slow sinus rate is seen between runs of atrial fibrillation or flutter. This is called the **tachycardia-bradycardia syndrome** because periods of rapid heart rate ("tachy") are separated by periods of slow heart rate ("brady"). Presumably, the absence of normal sinus activity makes it more likely that the atria will fibrillate or flutter (Fig. 12–18).

Unexplained phenomenon: Remember all those reserve pacemakers? They're supposed to turn on to drive the heart when the sinus node fails; however, in the sick sinus syndrome the reserve pacemakers fail too, or at least they don't function adequately. That's why the patient has problems. Why do all the reserve pacing systems fail just because the sinus node is sick? Nobody really knows, but that's what happens. A better name for the sick sinus syndrome would be "total pacemaker failure."

How dangerous is the sick sinus syndrome? Not very. It's rare for the sick sinus syndrome to stop the heart long enough to threaten life. The symptoms can be annoying, however, and can even make it impossible to function normally.

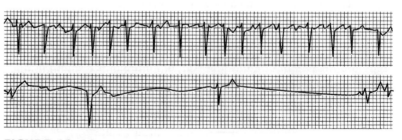

FIGURE 12–18

The top strip shows atrial fibrillation with a ventricular rate of about 110 bpm. In the bottom strip, the fibrillation has stopped and there is a very slow sinus rhythm with pauses of 3 seconds between beats. This is the "tachycardia-bradycardia" type of sick sinus syndrome, when a rapid atrial arrhythmia alternates with a slow sinus rhythm.

The sick sinus syndrome, therefore, is defined by symptoms. If a slow sinus rate causes significant symptoms, the sick sinus syndrome is present and treatment is justified. If there are no symptoms, the syndrome isn't present no matter how slow the sinus rate is.

How common is the sick sinus syndrome? As a matter of fact, it is very rare, although you may hear such statements as "But I know lots of people with pacemakers for the sick sinus syndrome," and "My doctor said it's the most common reason for having a pacemaker. It can't be all that rare." Oh, yes, it can. Real sick sinus is rare. False sick sinus is common. *False sick sinus?* Certainly.

The sinus node is extremely sensitive to a great many strong medications. Digitalis, quinidine, calcium-blocking drugs, beta-blocking drugs, clonidine, most of the drugs used to control hypertension, drugs used to control mental disturbances—this is a partial list of the medications that can slow the sinus node so much, it looks as though there's a true sick sinus syndrome.

The vagus nerve has a powerful depressing effect on the sinus node. Severe nausea and retching will stimulate the vagus nerve and slow the sinus node, often dramatically. Morphine and other pain-relieving drugs turn on the vagus nerve and often depress the sinus node. A bad hangover or a case of food poisoning can produce false sick sinus syndrome with alarming slowing of the heart rate.

Note: Far and away, the most common cause of false sick sinus syndrome is the administration of toxic drugs by physicians who are not familiar with the effect these drugs can have on the sinus node.

Treatment

The only treatment for true sick sinus syndrome is a pacemaker. In the brady-tachy form it may be necessary to give suppressive drugs like digitalis, quinidine, or procainamide after the pacemaker is implanted.

Note: There is never any urgency about implanting a permanent pacemaker. If sick sinus syndrome is suspected and if symptoms are severe, a temporary pacemaker can be implanted while the physician makes completely sure that drugs aren't the cause of the slow sinus rate. The patient should always insist on consultation by an outside expert and should always be sure that the physician has ruled out false sick sinus before a pacemaker is implanted.

ATRIOVENTRICULAR BLOCK

Here the trouble lies farther down the circuit. The activation impulse is formed normally in the sinus node and follows a normal track across the atria. The problem lies in the conducting tissues between atria and ventricles; they may be depressed, or they may not be able to function at all. This failure to function can take one of three forms.

1. The activating impulse may take longer than normal to reach the ventricles. Instead of 0.20 second, the PR may stretch out to 0.24, 0.28, or even to extreme lengths such as 0.60 second (Fig. 12–19). In other words, in this kind of atrioventricular block, every activating impulse does reach the ventricles—it just takes longer than normal doing it. This is **first-degree heart block**.

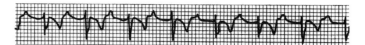

FIGURE 12–19
Normal sinus rhythm with first-degree heart block. The PR interval is over 0.20 second.

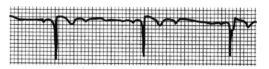

FIGURE 12–20
2:1 AV block. Every other P wave reaches the ventricles and produces a beat. The cells of the AV node take an abnormally long time to recover after transmitting this beat, and they aren't ready to conduct when the second P wave comes along. It's blocked. This period of block gives the AV nodal cells a chance to recover, and they're ready to conduct again when the third P wave appears.

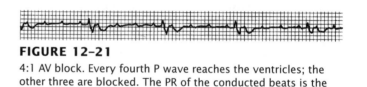

FIGURE 12–21
4:1 AV block. Every fourth P wave reaches the ventricles; the other three are blocked. The PR of the conducted beats is the same.

2. Some of the waves may reach the ventricles, while others are completely blocked and never get there. This is called **second-degree heart block;** it takes several forms.

   • **2:1 Heart block**—The diseased conducting tissues take a long time to recover after each transmission. As a result, they can't transmit very fast. It's common to see that only every other P wave is conducted. The alternate P wave runs into tissue that's refractory (unable to conduct because of fatigue) and never reaches the ventricles (Fig. 12–20). There may be other ratios—3:1 or higher—depending on how long it takes the tissues to recover after each transmission (Fig. 12–21).

   • **Wenckebach heart block**—This is a long name, but it's easy to remember; also important. In the atrioventricular node, you can imagine sick or poisoned cells acting like a line of workers with the flu. Suppose that these workers have to pass heavy cement blocks along the line many times a minute. The problem is that the workers are sick and very tired, so they take longer and longer to pass each block. Finally they all collapse and the next time the boss hands them a block, they tell him what to do with it. The block doesn't get passed. The pause gives the workers a rest and the next block that comes along is passed briskly, starting the whole cycle over. This is also called *type I block*. It's typical of the way cells in the AV node act when they're depressed (Figs. 12–22 and 12–23).

   • **Mobitz II block**—Before I can describe this type of block, it's important to talk about the bundle branches. Sometimes one bundle branch fails to conduct—usually because the cells in the bundle branch are diseased.

That's not a disaster because the other bundle branch can activate both ventricles perfectly well. It will take longer for the activating impulse to travel through the ventricles, but it's only a difference of a few hundredths of a second and it doesn't affect the pumping action of the heart.

The impulse comes down the normal bundle branch fast—4 meters per second. The impulse then has to enter the blocked ventricle "backward," slowly, like a car on a detour at about 0.5 meter per second (1/8 as fast as normal) (Fig. 12–24).

Since the ventricle takes longer than normal to be activated, the QRS will be wide—0.12 second or more. Thus, if a beat is conducted down from the atria and if the ventricular complex of that beat is 0.12 second wide, one bundle branch must be blocked.

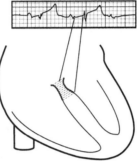

FIGURE 12–22
The Wenckebach type of AV block. The PR interval of the first beat is at the upper limits of normal (0.20 second). The second PR is much longer (0.32 second), and the third P wave is blocked. This cycle demonstrates the increasing fatigue of the diseased AV nodal cells until they completely refuse to transmit. After a rest period, the cycle starts over.

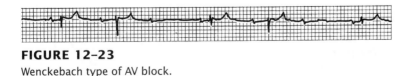

FIGURE 12–23
Wenckebach type of AV block.

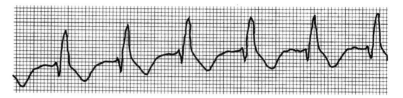

FIGURE 12–24

Bundle branch block. There is a sinus rhythm with a small P wave at a normal distance from each QRS. The QRS is wide (0.14 second), meaning that one bundle branch is blocked, and the activating impulse has to take a detour as it travels backward through the blocked ventricle.

In other words, if you can count to three, you can diagnose bundle branch block (three squares = 0.12 second).

If one bundle branch is permanently out, conduction from atria to ventricles depends on the other bundle branch. If that bundle branch fails to conduct occasionally, the dangerous form of block called **type II second-degree block**, or **Mobitz II block**, is present. This kind of block has a typical pattern in the electrocardiogram

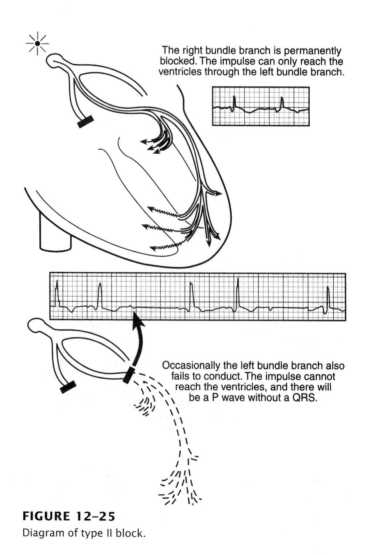

The right bundle branch is permanently blocked. The impulse can only reach the ventricles through the left bundle branch.

Occasionally the left bundle branch also fails to conduct. The impulse cannot reach the ventricles, and there will be a P wave without a QRS.

FIGURE 12–25

Diagram of type II block.

quite different from type I block. Suddenly, with no warning, one P wave isn't conducted. There isn't any change in the PR interval before or after the blocked P wave. Everything stays the same except that one or more impulses don't reach the ventricle. To make the diagnosis, the physician has to see that the PR interval stays the same in two or more consecutive beats—in other words, that there's no Wenckebach effect.

DIAGNOSIS OF MOBITZ II BLOCK

Figure 12-25 illustrates the electrocardiographic pattern of Mobitz II block. Type II block is very dangerous. Patients with this type of block have a 30% per year risk of a catastrophe when the heart stops beating. The shocking fact that I have learned in years of lecturing on this subject is that most physicians, including many prominent cardiologists, don't know how to distinguish type I block from type II. Here's why the distinction is so important. **Type I block is practically always located in the AV node**. It's often caused by drugs like digitalis, calcium blockers, or beta blockers. Stopping the drug is all that's needed to cure the block. It often comes on temporarily during myocardial infarcts involving the right coronary artery. When it does, it always goes away and no permanent treatment is needed. It's often seen as a normal variant in healthy young people, particularly during sleep, and these cases don't need any treatment at all.

Type II block is practically always located down in the bundle branches. It can only happen when one bundle branch is permanently out and the other fails now and then. It is very dangerous and often progresses to higher degrees of block. Permanent pacing is almost always necessary.

COMPLETE HEART BLOCK

The door between atria to ventricles is nailed shut. Nothing can pass from the top of the heart to the bottom. This is the time those ectopic pacemakers do what they're supposed to do—namely, save the patient's life. An ectopic pacemaker in the node or the ventricles begins a steady discharge and maintains a heartbeat. If it didn't, the patient would die (Fig. 12–26).

There are three criteria for the diagnosis of complete heart block: First, there is no electric connection between the atria and the ventricles. The atria are driven by the sinus node and the ventricles are driven by an ectopic pacemaker lower down. The two rhythms are completely independent. They are dissociated, to use the technical term.

Second, the rate of the ectopic pacemaker driving the ventricles is very slow. There is plenty of time between ectopic beats to let a normal beat come down if it could, but it never does. (A rate of 45 beats or less is accepted as slow enough to establish the diagnosis.)

Third, there are plenty of atrial complexes struggling to come through in the interval between the ectopic beats, but none of them do.

When all these conditions are met, complete heart block is present.

Complete heart block may be caused by total failure of conduction in the AV node (Fig. 12–27). It may also be caused by total failure of both bundle branches (Fig. 12–28).

Complete heart block caused by failure of both bundle branches is by far the more serious of the two forms. Permanent pacing is practically always required. Complete heart block caused by failure of the AV node is much less serious: it is often caused by

The sinoatrial node discharges normally, inscribing regular P waves, but all sinus impulses are blocked at the atrioventricular node.

Thus, ventricular rhythm is maintained by an ectopic focus in the lower atrioventricular node, the His bundle, or the ventricles.

As a result, P waves and ventricular complexes are disposed and superimposed at random with no consistent relationship to each other in ECG.

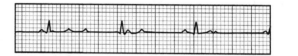

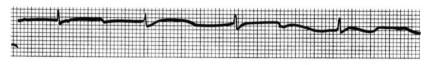

FIGURE 12–26
Complete AV block.

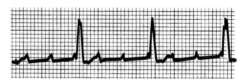

FIGURE 12–27
Complete heart block in the AV node. The narrow QRS complexes mean that the bundle branch system is functioning normally. The P waves are wandering through the tracing with no relationship to the QRS complexes. Life is maintained by an ectopic focus in the AV node.

FIGURE 12–28
Complete heart block caused by failure of both bundle branches. The ectopic focus driving the heart is in the ventricles, hence the typical wide, bizarre QRST complexes.

drugs or by temporary conditions that will be expected to improve. It's safe to say that 90% of cases of complete heart block localized in the AV node are caused by some factor outside the heart—drugs, myocardial infarction involving the right coronary artery, abnormalities of minerals in the blood, and so on. Any competent physician will go to great lengths to rule out these causes before recommending permanent pacing.

Commandments About Pacing for Complete Heart Block

If the complete AV block is permanent, and

If it is not caused by some drug that could be stopped, and

If it is not caused by some disease process that is predictably going to get better,

Then and only then, permanent pacing is necessary.

The conscientious physician and the intelligent patient will go to great lengths to make sure all these precautions are observed. A pacemaker inserted for the right reason can save a life; an unnecessary pacemaker can be a tragic event.

FATAL ARRHYTHMIAS: SUDDEN CARDIAC DEATH—VENTRICULAR FIBRILLATION

I remember an incident when I was a first lieutenant in the army medical corps. I was jogging at double time, when a cry and scuffle from the company behind halted the column. Stretched dead on the ground was a 35-year-old former bartender who had been in the service just 4 weeks. Why did the man die?

In accordance with army regulations a line-of-duty board was convened to decide whether the man's death had anything to do with his army service. (Since he left a widow, it was a foregone conclusion that we were going to find out it did.) The post-mortem examination showed one area of narrowing in the left anterior descending coronary artery—not very severe, and certainly not enough to cut down blood flow much. We were baffled at the time, but today the answer to the man's death is clear enough. The man died of ventricular fibrillation: a fatal disorder of heart rhythm. Cigarette smoking, mild obesity, total lack of physical conditioning, and sudden strenuous effort combined with a minor obstruction to blood flow to "short circuit" the normal flow of electric current across the ventricles and start the fine, fast, twitching motion that drops the victim like a shot (Fig. 12–29).

Remember atrial fibrillation? The atria stop their organized beating and begin a fine, fast, twitching motion that has been described as "like a can of worms." Fibrillation in the atria isn't an immediate danger since the atria don't do the real pumping of the blood. People can live for 20 or 30 years with fibrillating atria. When the ventricles fibrillate, on the other hand, no blood is pumped out of the heart and the victim falls instantly unconscious. The changes of death start within minutes.

There are two major categories of ventricular fibrillation. First, and most common, is ventricular fibrillation that occurs during myocardial infarction. If the heart isn't too badly damaged, the fibrillation can be stopped and a normal rhythm restored by electric shock. Some drugs are also helpful when used in conjunction with the electric shock. When ventricular fibrillation occurs as a complication of myocardial infarction, it isn't likely to recur. There's only about a 3% per year risk that it happens again.

On the other hand, when ventricular fibrillation comes "out of the blue," without an infarct or other obvious cause, there's a greatly increased chance it will happen again. In fact, the risk of another attack is about 30%.

Today this condition is always treated with an implanted defibrillator. These remarkable devices contain an electrocardiographic sensor that can diagnose

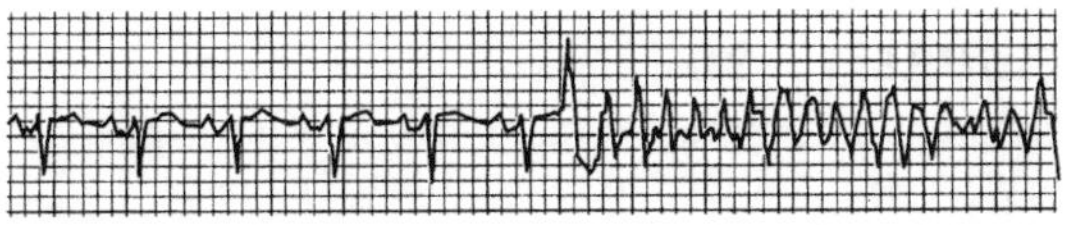

FIGURE 12–29
Onset of ventricular fibrillation, interrupting a normal sinus rhythm. A single ventricular ectopic beat acts as the trigger, and the ventricles go into the irregular, rapid twitching recorded in the ECG.

ventricular fibrillation and a shocking device exactly like the ones available in emergency rooms. It delivers a defibrillating shock that is very effective. Certainly anyone who has suffered an episode of ventricular fibrillation outside the setting of a myocardial infarction should have one of these devices implanted.

One test sometimes used in this setting is a study to see if the patient is "inducible." With defibrillating apparatus in place the patient is actually thrown into ventricular fibrillation and then cardioverted back to sinus rhythm. This is supposed to designate the patients at risk, but careful review has shown that it's not a very accurate test. There are other and better criteria for inserting defibrillators, as listed at the end of this chapter. (More about implanted defibrillators under the heading "Invasive Treatment of Arrhythmias" later in this chapter.)

TORSADE

In recent years physicians have learned to recognize a deadly arrhythmia that lies somewhere between ventricular tachycardia and ventricular fibrillation. It starts out with wide complexes like any ventricular tachycardia, but the shape and direction of these complexes then changes wildly. The direction of the complexes changes progressively from up to down and back again, as if the QRS were twisting around a wire. A French cardiologist compared this to a ballerina twisting on her toes, and came up with the name **torsades de pointes**—the name dancers use to describe this maneuver (Fig. 12–30). Torsade is often caused by drugs that prolong the interval from the beginning of the QRS to the end of the T wave: the QT interval. Quinidine and procainamide are the worst offenders, but all the newer drugs used to supress ventricular arrhythmias, such as sotalol and flecainide, carry about the same risk. Even amiodarone, the most commonly used drug for several arrhythmias, can cause this potentially lethal disorder. Sometimes it happens even when the QT interval is normal.

Torsade can be fatal, or it can be brief, producing no more than dizziness. Treatment is completely different from that for the other ventricular arrhythmias; the commonly used drugs are ineffective or may even make torsade worse. Intravenous magnesium is very effective. When this doesn't work, torsade can be stopped and recurrences can be prevented by pacing the heart rapidly from the atrium.

Increasing the heart rate, in other words, is an excellent way to stop torsade. The much-publicized sudden deaths of athletes are the result of ventricular fibrillation, torsade, or standstill. Proper cardiopulmonary resuscitation would save the great

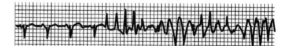

FIGURE 12–30

Torsades de pointes. A rapid ectopic ventricular rhythm starts after the fourth beat. The wide complexes change direction completely, from straight up to straight down and back again, like a ballerina twisting *sur les pointes* (on the points) of her ballet shoes. This is a dangerous variation of ventricular tachycardia and can lead to sudden cardiac death.

majority. Sometimes these deaths are associated with abnormalities of heart structure that go undetected on ordinary examination. Thickening of the muscle of the interventricular septum, or asymmetrical septal hypertrophy, is the commonest of these dangerous inborn deformities.

VENTRICULAR STANDSTILL

The name describes what happens—the heart stops beating and hangs perfectly still. No blood is pumped, and the results are the same as in ventricular fibrillation. Electric shock is no help in these cases; injection of various drugs sometimes restores a beat. Rarely, a pacemaker is helpful. Ventricular standstill is about 10 times as dangerous as ventricular fibrillation. It can be caused by coronary artery disease with massive infarction or by poisoning by various elements—for example, too much potassium (Fig. 12–31).

After resuscitation, what? Remember the key fact noted above: if a patient suffers sudden cardiac death in the course of a myocardial infarct, there isn't much danger of a recurrence. The risk is no more than 3% per year, and no special measures are needed. If sudden cardiac death occurs as an isolated event, the risk of recurrence is high—about 30% per year. Because of this very high risk of another fatal attack, the implantable pacemaker-defibrillator has been developed, and it's one of the great advances of recent years.

Electrodes are attached to the heart and a sensing device is implanted that combines a recording electrocardiogram with a pacemaker and a defibrillating device. The circuitry is incredibly sophisticated but the overall result is simple and often lifesaving.

First, if the heart stops beating or if the heart rate falls so low as to be dangerous, the pacemaker turns on and drives the heart.

Second, if the heart goes into ventricular fibrillation, the machine detects it at once and fires a defibrillating shock (Fig. 12–32).

The circuitry has improved dramatically in the last decade, and there have been numerous studies about which drugs to use to cut down the likelihood of ventricular fibrillation and the need for the lifesaving shock. (Patients will usually state that defibrillation "feels like being kicked by a horse." It's desirable to cut down the frequency of

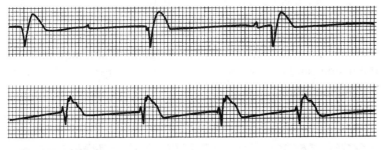

FIGURE 12–31
Events leading to standstill. In the top strip there is complete block with a very slow sinus rate (about 22 bpm) and a slow, independent ventricular rate of 32 bpm. In the bottom strip, there is no atrial activity. The very wide ventricular ectopic beats appearing at a rate of 43 bpm are characteristic of a dying heart that is barely twitching. After the last beat recorded on this strip, the heart stopped.

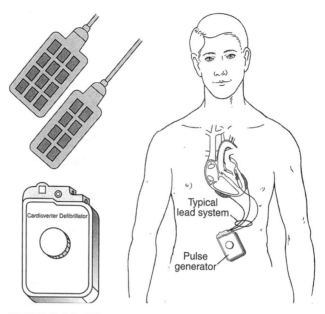

FIGURE 12-32
Implantable cardioventricular defibrillator.

shocks, even though they're lifesaving.) Probably amiodarone emerges as the best drug in this setting.

Speaking of amiodarone, it is essential to emphasize that *amiodarone alone does not prolong life in this setting, and that implantable defibrillators do.* Amiodarone may, however, cut down the frequency of defibrillating shocks, although this is still the subject of study.

Who needs one of these remarkable instruments?

First, certainly anyone who has suffered a cardiac arrest outside the setting of a myocardial infarct will benefit from an implantable defibrillator.

Second, anyone with one of the congenital sudden-death syndromes described in Chapter 12 would benefit from a defibrillator. (Since these diseases are genetic, a careful review of family history is essential.)

Third, new data suggest that anyone with critically depressed left ventricular function from coronary disease or some other cardiomyopathy may benefit from a defibrillator.

Finally, benefit for this last group may be better defined by testing for "inducibility"—that is, testing to see if ventricular fibrillation can be provoked in the laboratory. This is still a subject of debate and study. Medicare standards in this regard are very liberal, since an implantable defibrillator in most patients with severely depressed left ventricular function can be shown to be cost-effective in terms of lives saved and subsequent medical expenses.

CARDIOPULMONARY RESUSCITATION

We all stood around the unfortunate bartender and decided he was dead. We didn't know what else to do—but then neither did anybody else. Now we could probably save his life. Modern resuscitation with closed-chest massage is saving lives all over the civilized world. My colleagues Drs. Ewy and Kern here at the University of Arizona are pioneers in the technique of this kind of resuscitation and their work has "rewritten the book" on how to go about it. It's described at length in Chapter 22.

We do progress. Cardiopulmonary resuscitation, electric conversion of arrhythmias, and a useful battery of new drugs have made it possible to save many thousands of lives that would have been lost a generation ago.

INVASIVE TREATMENT OF CARDIAC ARRHYTHMIAS

Invasive treatment of cardiac arrhythmias has worked out surprisingly well in some specifically defined categories.

Supraventricular Tachycardia of the AV Nodal Reentrant Type

This constitutes about 98% of all supraventricular tachycardias and we now understand the mechanism. There are two tracts through the AV node, separated completely from each other as if they were little insulated wires. One of these tracts conducts rapidly, the other more slowly. AV nodal tachycardia is almost always caused by an impulse that goes down one nodal tract and back up the other in a self-perpetuating circuit. Depending on which tract conducts down and which back up, the electrophysiologist will refer to "slow-fast" or "fast-slow" tachycardia. The amazing fact is that a skilled electrophysiologist can introduce a wire into the nodal region, isolate one of the tracts and destroy it by radio frequency, thus eliminating the "up-down" tachycardia permanently.

Atrial Ectopic Tachycardia

This is a much rarer form of supraventricular tachycardia. It arises from a specific spot or focus somewhere above the atrioventricular node—that is, in the atria of the tissues immediately around them. The electrophysiologist has to catch the patient while the arrhythmia is actually going, map the location accurately, and then destroy it by radio frequency energy.

Ventricular Tachycardia

Many approaches have been tried for treating ventricular tachycardia. These usually include mapping the reentry loop or "track" of the tachycardia and then cutting an obstacle across it. Some successes have been achieved in this field, but the results aren't as good as with supraventricular tachycardias.

Atrial Flutter

Electrophysiologic study has revealed that many cases of flutter are caused by a counterclockwise circuit in the right atrium. This circuit depends on a particular area—the "isthmus" between the inferior vena cava and the tricuspid valve—to maintain itself. By cutting this isthmus with radio frequency energy, the electrophysiologist can cure the flutter permanently. The mechanism of flutter varies, and some types cannot be cured by this method, but all cases of recurrent flutter should be studied with this procedure in mind.

Atrial Fibrillation

Invasive treatment in this setting is still in the realm of experiment. Some brilliant French cardiologists discovered that atrial fibrillation is caused by atrial premature beats, usually originating in a pulmonary vein. (Remember, the pulmonary veins drain the blood from the lungs into the left atrium.) It's possible to stop recurrences of atrial fibrillation by "cutting" an area around the exit of the pulmonary veins by radio frequency so that the electric impulses of the premature beats can't reach the atria. Premature atrial beats leading to atrial fibrillation have been demonstrated in other parts of the left atrium: radio frequency can also be applied in these areas, with some success. Unfortunately, there have been serious complications with this method. The pulmonary vein may close off after the radio frequency has been applied, and there have been actual perforations of the left atrium with rupture into the esophagus. Both of these are obviously very serious, life-threatening complications; it's fair to say that this method is in need of further study. After all, atrial fibrillation is not a life-threatening arrhythmia: it doesn't seem reasonable to put a patient's life at risk in an attempt to cure it.

NOTES FOR CRITICAL CARE PERSONNEL

Figure 12–33 illustrates a harmless arrhythmia that's often confused with significant disorders: the wandering pacemaker. Note that the P waves change from inverted to upright and back again. They're perfectly regular, however, and there are no premature beats. The pacemaker is simply wandering around the sinoatrial node and down toward the AV node a little. This should never be confused with sick sinus syndrome. It's a variant of normal and doesn't call for any treatment.

An example of aberrant conduction is shown in Figure 12–34. The word **aberrant** comes from the latin *aberrare*, "to go astray." Aberrant conduction simply means abnormally low conduction—usually in some part of the ventricular network. Aberrant conduction takes place when some part of the conducting network takes too long to recover from the previous transmission. In other words, the refractory period is prolonged. As a result, the next activating wave finds some part of the network unable to conduct and has to go around a "detour." Bundle branch block is the ultimate form of aberrancy. In Figure 12–34 the third, fifth, and seventh beats are premature atrial beats interrupting a normal sinus rhythm. Note the very prominent "spiky" P wave in the premature beats. These beats arrive so early that they find a part of the ventricular

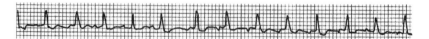

FIGURE 12–33
ECG tracing of a harmless arrhythmia often mistaken for a pathologic one.

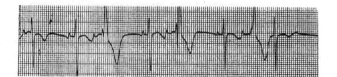

FIGURE 12–34
Aberrant conduction.

conducting system refractory and so they are conducted aberrantly, with a wide, bizarre QRST complex.

Aberrant conduction can be quite confusing (Fig. 12–35). The basic rhythm is atrial fibrillation: during the brief pauses the characteristic f waves of coarse atrial fibrillation are obvious. When the rate slows, the QRS is normal—note the first beat in the top strip and the two narrow beats in the middle of the bottom strip. When conduction to the ventricles speeds up, the QRS complexes become wide because of rate-dependent bundle branch block, the extreme form of aberrancy. One bundle branch has a prolonged refractory period and simply cannot conduct above a certain rate. This kind of aberrancy can be confused with ventricular tachycardia, but the clues here are the appearance of narrow complexes when the rate slows, the grossly irregular rhythm, and the obvious fibrillary waves.

All this leads up to Figure 12–36, which shows a wide-beat tachycardia without visible P waves. This might be a junctional tachycardia with bundle branch block or it might be ventricular tachycardia—**from an ECG like this, it's not possible to make the distinction with acceptable accuracy**. There are some criteria (dissociated atrial rhythm, capture beats with fusion, certain types of morphology of the QRS) that make it very likely that a wide-beat tachycardia is ventricular.

On the other hand, there is no way of saying with acceptable accuracy that a particular wide-beat tachycardia is *not* ventricular. There are no criteria that permit the observer to say that aberrant conduction is the cause of the wide-beat tachycardia with an accuracy of more than 80% to 85%, and that's not good enough for a life-threatening arrhythmia.

What does this mean to the patient? How does all this influence treatment?

The reasoning is simple. The drugs used for ventricular tachycardia are amiodrarone, procainamide, and lidocaine. (There are many others but they're not as effective.) If the wide-beat tachycardia is really junctional rather than ventricular, those won't do any harm and the amiodrarone and procainamide may be effective.

On the other hand, the agents used for supraventricular tachycardia—digitalis or verapamil—may be lethal if the rhythm is really ventricular tachycardia.

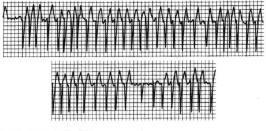

FIGURE 12–35
Confusing aberrant conduction.

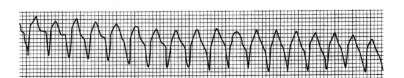

FIGURE 12–36
Wide-beat tachycardia.

The game of looking at a wide-beat tachycardia and deciding that it "looks like aberrancy" is a form of Russian roulette.

The rule is simple: *In the presence of a wide-beat tachycardia, always treat for the more dangerous possibility—that is, for ventricular tachycardia. Critical care personnel should never be put in the position of trying to make the distinction between the two types of wide-beat tachycardia; even highly skilled cardiologists often cannot do it.*

Digitalis-Toxic Rhythms

An overdosage of digitalis can slow the heart rate by depressing the sinus node or delaying conduction through the AV node.

When digitalis toxicity produces a rapid rate, diagnosis can be difficult. It is also critical; the digitalis-toxic tachyarrhythmias are very dangerous. The wrong treatment—that is, more digitalis—is likely to be fatal. Here are some simple rules:

1. *Always* assume that *any* paroxysmal tachycardia in a digitalized patient is caused by digitalis toxicity until proved otherwise. This is true whether the tachycardia arises in the atria, the AV node, or the ventricles.

2. Patients with chronic atrial fibrillation are almost always maintained on digitalis. When one of these patients presents with a rapid regular pulse, always see that an ECG is recorded and a diagnosis established promptly. The chances are overwhelming that a digitalis-toxic junctional tachycardia is present (Fig. 12–37). The top strip records typical atrial fibrillation; in the bottom strip, there is a rapid, regular rhythm with the same QRST configuration as in the conducted beats in the top strip. This is a junctional tachycardia, caused by digitalis toxicity. Rapid junctional rhythms are the commonest tachycardia produced by digitalis toxicity. Treatment: stop digitalis, give potassium, wait. In rare cases, antidigitalis antibodies may be needed.

3. Paroxysmal atrial tachycardia (PAT) with AV block is almost always produced by digitalis toxicity combined with a low-serum potassium. It can take many forms and it's often hard to recognize. Figure 12–38 shows a typical example of this disorder. The P waves are large and peaked and easy to recognize. The atrial rate is about 215 bpm and the atrial rhythm is perfectly regular. Some of the P waves reach the ventricles and produce beats, while some are blocked. The ratio of P waves to QRS complexes varies—2:1, 3:1, 4:1—so that the ventricular rhythm is completely irregular. It would be easy to confuse it with atrial fibrillation. More digitalis at this point would probably kill the patient. Treatment: potassium intravenously, rapidly—as much as 40 milliequivalent (mEq) in 2 hours, if needed.

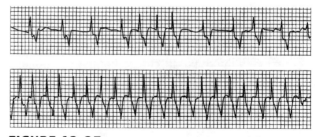

FIGURE 12–37
Digitalis-toxic junctional tachycardia.

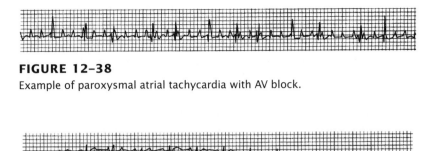

FIGURE 12–38
Example of paroxysmal atrial tachycardia with AV block.

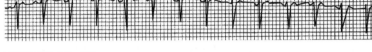

FIGURE 12–39
PAT with 2:1 block.

Note: Never treat a rapid, irregular rhythm until a definitive diagnosis has been established by an electrocardiogram.

Figure 12–39 shows just how tricky the diagnosis of PAT with block can be. Here the ventricular rhythm is slow and regular, with a rate of 98 bpm. Notice the extra P wave coming just after each QRS; the atrial rate is twice as fast as the ventricular rate. This is PAT with 2:1 block. It would be easy to mistake this for a simple sinus rhythm.

There is a specific treatment for digitalis-toxic ventricular tachycardia—diphenylhydantoin, or phenytoin. The effect is dramatic and consistent. It is given intravenously in 100-mg boluses every 5 minutes until the arrhythmia is stopped, or until 1 gram (g) has been given, or until neurologic complications appear. It usually doesn't take a very large dose to stop the arrhythmia.

Regarding the use of lidocaine soon after an infarct, refer to Appendix A.

SUDDEN DEATH, YOUR GRANDFATHER'S GENES, THE ECG, AND DEFIBRILLATORS

Since the last edition of this book we've learned a great deal about some inherited abnormalities that can cause sudden death. These dangerous entities can be recognized *only* through the electrocardiogram and they all involve the recovery period of the heart cycle, that is, the ST segment and the T wave. (Remember, this is the period when activation has been completed and the cells are beginning to start repolarization, or recovery of potential.)

For many years medical science has recorded two rare inherited disorders that can cause sudden death: (1) Jervell and Lange-Nielsen, and (2) Romano-Ward.

The Jervell and Lange-Nielsen syndrome combines congenital deafness, a prolonged QT interval, and sudden death. Previously, these patients never survived much beyond childhood.

The Romano-Ward syndrome is the same thing, without the deafness.

Early in the study of electrocardiography physicians learned that a prolonged interval between the beginning of the QRS complex and the end of the T wave (the QT interval) was a dangerous finding, often associated with sudden death, and these two inherited patterns simply underlined the problem. (Go back to Chap. 11 and look at Fig. 11–7 again so that you know what the QT interval means.)

Some brilliant Spanish cardiologists recognized another form of genetic abnormality in the resting-recovery phase of the heart cycle defined by the ST segment. Drs. Brugada, Brugada, and Brugada (yes, they're three brothers) described a syndrome that combines elevation of the ST segment in the leads recorded on the right precordium (the leads just right and left of the sternum) with a high risk of sudden death (Fig. 12-40).

Once this syndrome—called the Brugada syndrome—was recognized, physicians all over the world reported cases—especially in Southeast Asia and parts of Italy. (We've had a case here at the University of Arizona Medical Center.)

This peculiar elevation of ST segments may not always be present but it can be brought out by certain drugs, principally procaine amide and ajmaline. (This latter drug is not yet available in the United States, although it's widely used in Europe and elsewhere. Someone needs to nudge the Food and Drug Administration because it's a safe and useful agent.)

When a person reports "passing out" with no obvious cause, the informed cardiologist will always test for the Brugada syndrome. Implantation of a defibrillator is the only treatment, and it's urgent.

These same remarkable brothers also detected another inherited syndrome that can cause sudden death; astonishingly, it's the *short* QT syndrome! Again, a genetic abnormality in the resting-recovery or ST–T portion of the heart cycle predisposes to ventricular fibrillation in apparently normal people. There's a table of QT intervals related to rate and sex in Appendix C. As a general rule, "short" means something less than 30 seconds.

Before deciding that one of these syndromes is present, of course, the intelligent cardiologist will rule out other causes of change in the QT interval. Elevation of serum calcium shortens the QT, whereas a low calcium level prolongs it: so do many drugs.

These are all basically syndromes recognized by the ECG only. Does invasive electrophysiologic study help in detecting these syndromes? The subject is hotly debated today. Remember, invasive electrophysiologic study here means actually

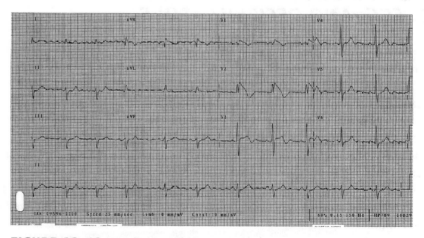

FIGURE 12–40

Brugada's Syndrome. Note the bizarre elevation of the ST segments in the right precordial leads—leads V1,2, andd 3. This is the characteristic finding and indiciates a high likelihood of sudden death. The only treatment is an implantable defibrillator. (To everyone's surprise, the older drug quinidine is helpful. It isn't a substitute for a defibrillator but it apparently cut down on the number of shocks.)

shocking the heart to see if it goes into ventricular fibrillation. It's not at all clear that this is helpful in this group of patients.

There's only one treatment for any of these syndromes, and that's an implantable defibrillator. Drugs are worthless.

Genetic testing is also helpful. The specific genes involved in these syndromes can be identified easily. Since these syndromes are heritable, it's essential to determine whether others in the family tree have been affected. (As usual, a careful medical history is the good right arm of diagnosis!)

These syndromes often appear in young people, so recognition and treatment are critical in terms of lives saved.

CHAPTER 13

Congenital Heart Disease

Why are some children born with abnormal hearts? Sometimes we can answer this agonizing question; sometimes we can't.

Certain infections during early fetal life can produce various types of birth deformities, including abnormalities of the heart structure. German measles is a familiar example. To some extent, these diseases and the abnormalities that go with them are preventable.

Some abnormal genes, like the gene of Down syndrome, carry abnormality of the heart structure encoded right on the DNA that determines everything about us. At our present stage of medical knowledge, there's no way of preventing these complications.

Many congenital heart abnormalities simply appear for no reason in otherwise healthy individuals.

About 1 out of every 1,000 babies born will have a congenital heart defect. Because of the early death of the more severe cases, about 1 in 3,000 will have an abnormal heart at the end of 1 year of life.

Parents who have one child with congenital heart disease have a slightly increased risk of the same kind of disease in a second child. The word *slightly* is emphasized here—the difference in risk isn't very great.

This chapter discusses the major forms of congenital heart disease in their order of occurrence.

CONGENITAL AORTIC STENOSIS

In the Western world today, most aortic stenosis is congenital; the acquired type associated with rheumatic fever has become rare. The disease starts with an abnormally constructed aortic valve. Instead of the normal three-valve flaps, this valve has only two—hence the term **bicuspid aortic valve** (Fig. 13–1).

The two-flap valve by itself isn't a problem, but in some cases the tissue of the valve is thickened and rigid at birth and the aortic opening is very narrow. The usual complications of aortic stenosis will follow: congestive heart failure, dizziness, and fainting. In severe cases, the only treatment is surgery, and the results are good.

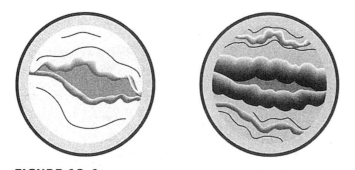

FIGURE 13-1
Bicuspid aortic valve in congenital aortic stenosis.

The great majority of bicuspid valves don't present any problem in early life, but in later years 50% of these valves will calcify and narrow, with significant aortic stenosis.

The symptoms are those to be expected when the entire blood supply for the body has to force its way through a narrow slit. Dizziness, fainting, angina pectoris, and congestive heart failure are all common manifestations. The risk of sudden death is very high after symptoms appear, and the only treatment is surgery. Once symptoms have appeared, there is no excuse for delay.

SEPTAL DEFECTS

Remember that there isn't supposed to be any connection between the two sides of the heart. Sometimes during fetal development, there's a failure of closure of the septum between the two sides of the heart and the child is born with a gap, or defect, in the septum. The defect—it's really just a hole—may lie between either the atria or the ventricles. The ventricular type is more common.

Ventricular Septal Defects

The pressure in the left ventricle is about five times as high as the pressure in the right throughout systole. If there is a hole in the septum between the ventricles, blood will flow from the left ventricle to the right, into the lungs, and back around to the left ventricle (Fig. 13–2).

If the hole is small, this isn't important. The heart can accommodate a small extra volume of blood going around the circuit and the patient can live a normal life.

If the hole is large, there is real danger. Now there is a large volume of blood being pumped into the lungs with a rapid, turbulent flow. The blood vessels of the lungs are fragile, not made to stand this kind of pressure and flow. Over the years they harden, with thickening of the coats of the small arteries (Fig. 13–3). This hardening of the pulmonary arteries causes the pressure in the pulmonary vessels to rise. Finally, the pressure in the pulmonary vessels may be as high as the pressure in the aorta.

At this point, the flow of blood will reverse, right to left, because the high pressure in the right ventricle will force some blood through the defect into the left ventricle. The patient will turn cyanotic (blue) because of the appearance in the arteries of unoxygenated blood that didn't go through the lungs. This is called the

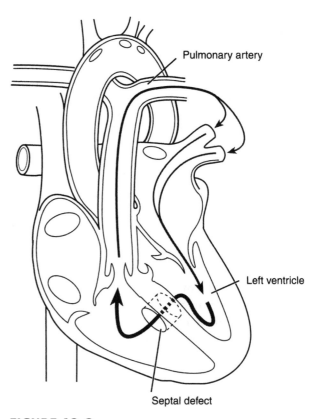

Pulmonary artery

Left ventricle

Septal defect

FIGURE 13–2

Ventricular septal defect. Some blood flows through the septal defect from the left ventricle to the right ventricle and back around through the lungs to the left ventricle again. Blood flows from the left atrium to the left ventricle. Some blood flows through the ventricular septal defect in the right ventricle. This shunted blood then flows out through the pulmonary artery and back to the left ventricle.

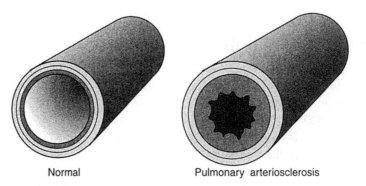

Normal   Pulmonary arteriosclerosis

FIGURE 13–3

(*Left*) Normal pulmonary artery. (*Right*) High pressure and rapid flow of blood into the small pulmonary arteries causes them to thicken—pulmonary arteriosclerosis takes place. It cannot be reversed.

Eisenmenger phenomenon (Fig. 13–4). When this happens, there's nothing to be done for the disease.

On the other hand, it's easy to close a ventricular septal defect surgically. If it is closed in time, the reaction in the lungs will not take place and the patient will be able to live a normal life, with no bad effects.

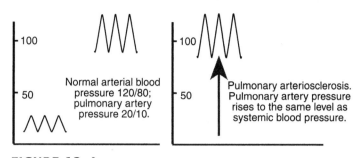

FIGURE 13–4
The Eisenmenger phenomenon.

Note: Ventricular septal defects of any size should be closed surgically before this fatal reaction takes place.

Any child with a ventricular septal defect should be studied very carefully to check the size of the defect.

Atrial Septal Defects

There are some interesting differences between atrial septal defects and those in the ventricular septum.

When an atrial septal defect is present, the blood flows through the hole from the left atrium to the right atrium, then to the right ventricle and pulmonary artery. The extra blood never reaches the left ventricle; it flows through the defect from left atrium to right before it gets there. There's no fluid load on the left side of the heart (Fig. 13–5).

Even though the volume of blood flowing through the defect may be large, it doesn't affect the small pulmonary arteries the way a ventricular septal defect does. Atrial septal defect is not nearly as dangerous as a ventricular septal defect because the Eisenmenger reaction is very rare with atrial defects. The reason for this difference is probably the low velocity of the blood moving through the atrial shunt and into the lungs, as well as the absence of turbulence in the flow.

With an interatrial septal defect of the common kind, there are no symptoms until late middle age, when the pressure in the pulmonary artery may rise moderately. When pressures in the pulmonary artery reach the range of 60/40 instead of the normal 15/5, the patient will often feel some chest discomfort and may have trouble breathing. At this point, surgery is needed. Fortunately, it's not difficult, and the results are excellent.

Very rarely, a huge atrial septal defect will increase pulmonary artery pressure to the danger point. For this reason, any atrial septal defect should be studied carefully to assess its size and its effect on pulmonary artery pressure.

The common kind of atrial septal defect shown in Figure 13–6 consists of a hole in the atrial septum only. It is called a secundum type of atrial septal defect and it is relatively harmless.

A much rarer form of atrial septal defect extends down into the septum between the ventricles. This is more severe and often leads to the Eisenmenger reaction. It should always be repaired surgically as soon as the patient's condition permits. This is called a primum type of atrial septal defect (Fig. 13–7).

A competent cardiologist can detect an atrial septal defect and can distinguish between the two types in about 5 or 10 minutes of work with a stethoscope, an electrocardiogram, and a chest x-ray.

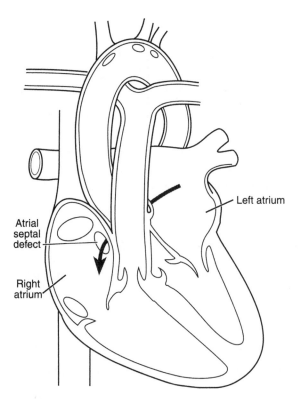

Left atrium

Atrial septal defect

Right atrium

FIGURE 13–5
Atrial septal defect. The arrow indicates the flow of blood from the left atrium (LA) to the right atrium (RA), thus overloading the right heart, pulmonary circulation, and left heart. There is no cyanosis because the blood shunts from the left to the right heart.

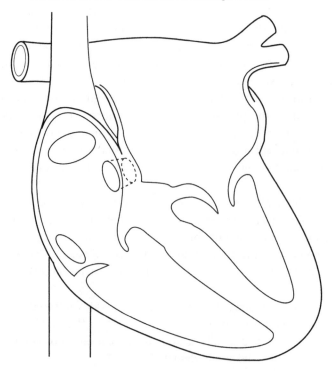

FIGURE 13–6
Ostium secundum atrial septal defect. This is a simple hole between the atria.

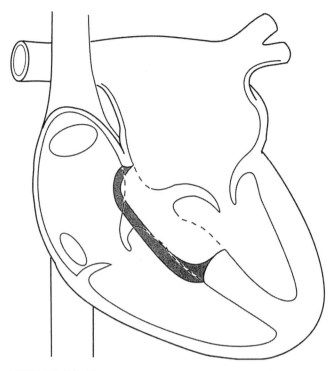

FIGURE 13–7
Ostium primum atrial septal defect. The hole extends down
into the septum between the ventricles.

PATENT DUCTUS ARTERIOSUS

A fetus can't breathe because it's floating in liquid. The mother breathes for it, and oxygen is carried to the fetus from the mother's circulation. A blood vessel from the placenta carries oxygenated blood to the baby's veins because the lungs aren't working yet. The blood is short-circuited around the lungs and delivered to the aorta by the channel called the ductus arteriosus (Fig. 13–8).

After birth, when the baby starts to breathe, the ductus isn't needed anymore, and in normal conditions it shrivels up and disappears in about 2 weeks. Sometimes it doesn't disappear, which creates a problem. If the ductus stays open, blood from the aorta is pumped into the pulmonary artery. This extra load of blood circulates back through the lungs and into the left ventricle before it starts back around the circuit (Fig. 13–9).

If the ductus is large, this extra load can wear down the left ventricle, leading to congestive heart failure. In later years, the high-velocity flow into the lungs can lead to an Eisenmenger reaction.

A small ductus arteriosus does not throw any significant load on the heart. In some premature infants, a small ductus can be induced to close by administration of the common antiinflammatory drug indomethacin. If a ductus is large enough to permit significant flow, surgical closure will always be necessary. Surgical closure of a patent ductus arteriosus is the easiest of all major heart operations since the heart itself doesn't have to be opened.

Note: Any persistent patent ductus arteriosus should be studied carefully by a competent cardiologist and surgery should be considered early. All the lethal complications can be prevented and the patient can look forward to a normal life.

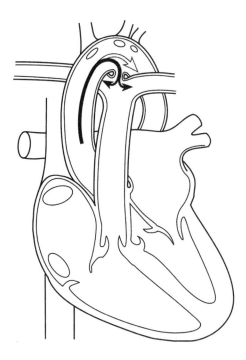

FIGURE 13–8
Patent ductus arteriosus. Flow of blood from the aorta through a patent ductus to the pulmonary artery causes overloading of the pulmonary circulation.

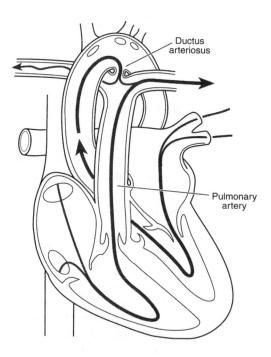

FIGURE 13–9
If the ductus stays open, blood flows through the ductus from the aorta to the pulmonary artery. This shunted blood flows back through the lungs to the left heart and out the aorta.

COARCTATION OF THE AORTA

Whenever hypertension turns up in a young patient, this congenital abnormality should be high on the list of possible causes. Coarctation of the aorta means that there's a narrowing of the aorta somewhere in the arch where it leaves the heart or sometimes a little lower down (Fig. 13–10).

This narrowing of the aorta naturally causes a high blood pressure above it and a low pressure below it, just like a dam in a stream. The blood pressure in the arms will be high and the blood pressure in the arteries of the legs and feet will be very low. It usually isn't possible to feel the pulses in the feet. The hypertension produced by the coarctation is just as dangerous as any hypertension—strokes, heart failure, and coronary episodes are the usual complications. Coarctation is easy to correct surgically because it isn't necessary to enter the heart. The narrow obstruction can be removed and a normal aortic channel restored at remarkably little risk to the patient. The combination of high blood pressure in the upper half of the body, low blood pressure in the lower half, and a characteristic heart murmur makes the diagnosis simple in the great majority of cases.

Bicuspid aortic valve and coarctation of the aorta are often found in combination. The coarctation practically always requires surgery; the bicuspid valve doesn't need treatment unless it becomes stenotic or regurgitant in later life.

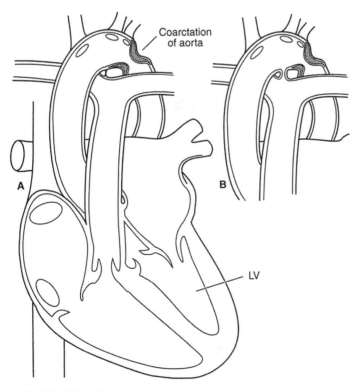

FIGURE 13–10
A. Coarctation of the aorta with normally closed ductus. The narrowing of the inside of the aorta puts a strain on the pumping left ventricle (LV). **B.** Coarctation of the aorta with patent ductus arteriosus.

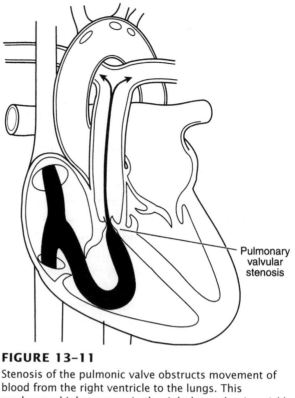

FIGURE 13–11
Stenosis of the pulmonic valve obstructs movement of
blood from the right ventricle to the lungs. This
produces a high pressure in the right heart that is quickly
transmitted back into the veins of the body. It also cuts
down blood flow to the lungs; this can be dangerous
during periods of increased oxygen demand, such as
while exercising.

PULMONIC VALVE STENOSIS

Congenital narrowing of the pulmonic valve is easy to recognize and relatively easy to
correct. Severe stenosis of the pulmonic valve cuts down blood flow to the lungs and
causes severe back pressure in the right heart and the veins of the body. In other
words, pulmonic stenosis causes "pure" right heart failure without any involvement of
the lungs or the left heart (Fig. 13–11). Dizziness and faintness on sudden exertion are
common with severe pulmonic stenosis. Subnormal blood flow to the lungs at a time of
greatly increased need is the cause. Teenagers often become aware of the symptoms
during athletic practice.

When symptoms appear, surgical correction is urgent—sudden death is common
with severe pulmonic stenosis.

TETRALOGY OF FALLOT

Imagine a combination of pulmonic stenosis with a ventricular septal defect—these are
the elements of the tetralogy of Fallot. The pulmonic stenosis produces a high pressure
in the right ventricle. As a result of this high pressure, blood flows through the ventricular septum from right to left. Unoxygenated dark venous blood is pumped into the left
ventricle and the arteries of the body. The patient turns blue, or cyanotic (Fig. 13–12).

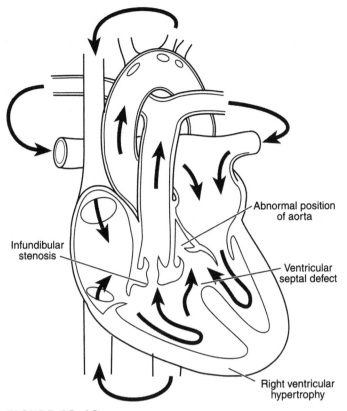

FIGURE 13–12
Tetralogy of Fallot. Because of the obstructing infundibular
pulmonary stenosis, blood flows through a ventricular septal
defect into the abnormally placed aorta. The right-to-left shunt
produces cyanosis.

There are many varieties of tetralogy, depending on the size of the opening in the
pulmonic valve and the size of the hole in the ventricular septum. If the pulmonic
stenosis isn't severe and if the septal defect is small, the patient may not suffer any significant effects. On the other hand, if the pulmonic stenosis is severe, with high pressures in the right ventricle, and if the septal defect is large, a great quantity of venous
blood will be pumped into the arteries and the patient will be in severe distress early
in life. Surgical correction of tetralogy is easy in competent hands and the long-term
results are excellent. Since there is no extra flow of blood into the lungs, there is never
an Eisenmenger effect, and the patient can resume normal life.
*Note: Any tetralogy should be precisely assessed by a skilled cardiologist who can make
decisions about timing of surgery.*

COMPLETE TRANSPOSITION
OF THE GREAT VESSELS

This is one of the most dangerous of congenital abnormalities. The good news is that it
can now be corrected surgically with excellent results.

The name of this abnormality tells the story. The aorta arises from the right ventricle and the pulmonary artery from the left. As a result, the blood from the veins
never reaches the lungs but is simply pumped from the right ventricle to the body. The
blood in the left ventricle is pumped in and out of the lungs through the wrong-sided

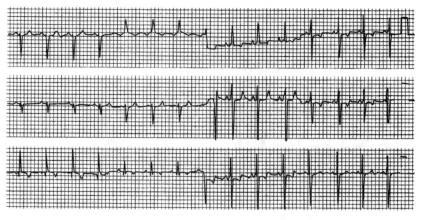

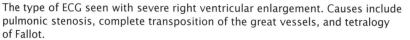

FIGURE 13–13
The type of ECG seen with severe right ventricular enlargement. Causes include pulmonic stenosis, complete transposition of the great vessels, and tetralogy of Fallot.

pulmonary artery, but it never moves forward to the body. Since the blood flowing through the arteries has never been through the lungs, it is dark, and the baby will have a bluish color, referred to as cyanosis. The electrocardiogram will have a typical configuration revealing the enormous pressure load on the right ventricles as it pumps against arterial pressures (Fig. 13–13).

Life isn't possible in this setting unless there is some connection between the aorta and the pulmonary artery to allow some venous blood to reach the lungs. The ductus arteriosus performs this function early in life, but it isn't enough. Surgical relief within hours or days is a matter of life and death.

The emergency operation for complete transposition is the Rashkind procedure. The arterial and venous circulations have to have a connection between them so that some blood can flow through the lungs and out to the body. This is done by creating an artificial atrial septal defect. A catheter is forced through the natural small hole between the atria called the foramen ovale. When this catheter is in the left atrium, a strong balloon at the end of it is inflated and the balloon is then pulled forcefully back into the right atrium, actually ripping a hole in the septum. It sounds brutal, but it works. The oxygenated blood from the left atrium now flows into the right atrium, right ventricle, and out the right-sided aorta to the body. This mixing saves the baby's life. In a few years the transposition can be completely corrected by the Mustard procedure, which reverses flow in the atria and makes normal circulation possible.

A lifetime as a physician holds some memories for which I must be truly grateful. One morning, in the heart laboratory in our hospital in Casper, Wyoming, our gifted chief technician, Betty Holmes, showed me an electrocardiogram.

"I took it on a newborn in the nursery just now," she said. "Dr. So-and-so said it was normal, but I don't think so. How about it?"

It was anything but normal. The ECG showed unmistakable signs of a huge right ventricle, a chamber that must be dangerously overloaded. I called the physician who was caring for the baby.

"Is the child cyanotic?" I asked.

"Blue as the midnight sky," he said.

"Complete transposition," I told him. "Needs surgery today."

Within 2 hours we had a plane ready to fly the child to Denver, thanks to the Crippled Children's Division of the State Health Department, and in 6 hours the lifesaving operation had been performed.

These are some of the commonest congenital abnormalities of the structure of the heart. A complete list would fill a large volume. There are some general comments on congenital heart disease that are important to anyone who has to deal with the disease.

ENDOCARDITIS

Endocarditis is a danger in any form of congenital heart disease except for the secundum type of atrial septal defect. When any other lesion is present, the patient must receive prophylactic antibiotics before, during, and after any surgical procedure—down to and including dental cleaning of the teeth. Patent ductus arteriosus and ventricular septal defect are especially dangerous lesions when it comes to infection.

ADVICE FOR PARENTS OF A CHILD WITH A CARDIAC DEFECT

Parents of a child with a congenital heart abnormality have to confront the problem of living with the disease. Here are a few useful principles.

1. Let the child find his or her own limits of physical exertion. It's common to see a child turn cyanotic while playing, suddenly stop and squat, turn pink again, and go on playing. The child is obeying natural feedback messages that tell him what to do. In the same way, a child will exert until he begins to feel shortness of breath and will then stop on his own accord. Children have better sense than adults; left to themselves they control their own activities very competently.

2. Don't make a permanent cardiac cripple out of the child. Most congenital heart diseases can be corrected surgically and the child should understand that the doctor can fix what's wrong even though it may be necessary to wait until the right age to do it. Don't force too much solicitude on the child and don't let your own anxiety show—it rubs off to a degree you can hardly imagine.

3. Remember that sudden cardiac death is rare in congenital heart disease. In this sense it's very different from coronary artery disease. The child may become short of breath, or go into frank congestive heart failure, but there's usually time to start medical management.

4. When the doctor or dentist prescribes endocarditis prophylaxis, **make sure the child takes the medication!**

Rheumatic Heart Disease

Rheumatic fever and rheumatic heart disease were major causes of death and disability throughout the world 50 years ago. Today, rheumatic fever is so rare in the United States and other westernized countries that whole generations of medical students are graduating without ever seeing a case. On the other hand, throughout the Third World—in Africa, Asia, and Latin America—rheumatic heart disease is common and virulent. In countries of the Eastern Mediterranean, Arab children sometimes progress to severe congestive heart failure from rheumatic heart disease by the age of 12. Even in the United States, the disease persists in remote areas and in isolated ethnic groups. Why have rheumatic fever and rheumatic heart disease disappeared from such a large part of the world? The answer is simple: **Rheumatic heart disease is completely preventable. It's the only kind of heart disease that is**.

RHEUMATIC FEVER: THE CAUSE AND CONSEQUENCES

Rheumatic fever is caused by the reaction of the body to a specific kind of germ—the group A beta-hemolytic streptococcus, or strep, as almost everyone knows it. It is caused by a specific kind of infection with this germ—the familiar "strep throat."

To understand what happens you have to know something about the way the body reacts to infections. The only reason you don't die when the first bacteria attack you is that the cells of your body have ways of resisting the bacteria by actually destroying them, and by neutralizing the toxic products they produce. This is called the immune reaction of the body. (In the H. G. Wells science fiction story that scared half the United States, a gang of Martians almost conquered the world until they were killed by bacteria; their bodies had no immune systems to fight off infection.)

Sometimes the immune system overreacts. The body goes on producing antidotes to the poisons of the bacteria long after the bacteria are gone. These **antibodies,** as they are called, actually become harmful to the tissues of the body and cause what is called **autoimmune disease**.

Imagine a company of soldiers defending a fort against invaders who keep coming over the walls. The soldiers kill all the invaders but become so trigger-happy that they keep blasting away, shooting holes in the fort itself and destroying the very structure they're supposed to be defending. This is what happens in autoimmune diseases, including rheumatoid arthritis, lupus erythematosis, rheumatic fever, and many others (Fig. 14–1).

The sequence of events in rheumatic fever goes like this. Day 1: A streptococcus attacks the throat, producing some signs or symptoms of infection. Days 4–5: With or without treatment, the sore throat gets better. Days 7–14: If the infection isn't treated with antibiotics, the rheumatic reaction will follow in one case out of a hundred or a thousand, depending on whether there's an epidemic going on and where the patient lives. Widespread inflammation starts in many parts of the body brought on by the immune reaction to the streptococcus. This reaction may attack the joints, the skin, the heart, the lungs and, later, the brain. After a few days, the inflammation in these tissues takes on a specific form called the Aschoff body. Each Aschoff body under the microscope looks like an adolescent pimple that never quite comes to a head but remains angry and red. There are millions of these microscopic sores and they keep recurring in new crops. This continuing inflammation can go on for many months.

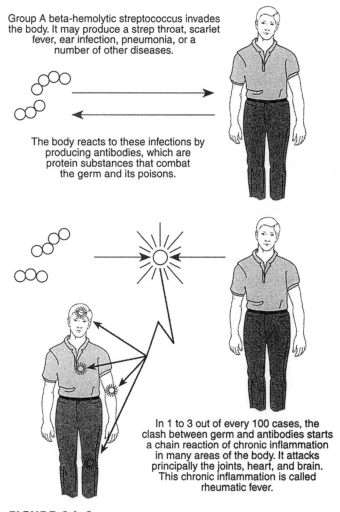

Group A beta-hemolytic streptococcus invades the body. It may produce a strep throat, scarlet fever, ear infection, pneumonia, or a number of other diseases.

The body reacts to these infections by producing antibodies, which are protein substances that combat the germ and its poisons.

In 1 to 3 out of every 100 cases, the clash between germ and antibodies starts a chain reaction of chronic inflammation in many areas of the body. It attacks principally the joints, heart, and brain. This chronic inflammation is called rheumatic fever.

FIGURE 14–1
Rheumatic fever reaction.

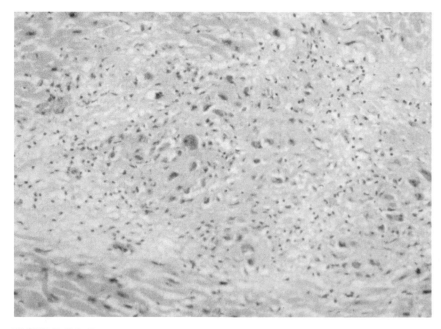

FIGURE 14-2

Aschoff body of rheumatic carditis. The more organized cells on the top and bottom are normal myocardial cells. The darker, rounded area in the center is of an Aschoff body, the basic lesion of rheumatic fever. It consists of a mass of various types of inflammatory cells and some surrounding scar tissue. (Courtesy of Dr. Richard E. Sobonya, Pathology Department, University of Arizona Medical Center.)

In the joints, it produces redness, swelling, and tenderness. In the skin, it produces a short-lived rash, called erythema marginatum, that's gone in a day or two. In the lungs, the inflammation can produce pneumonitis, or inflammation of lung tissue. In the brain, as a late complication, it can produce chorea, or St. Vitus' dance. None of these reactions are serious. They all go away with no serious aftereffects.

What *is* serious is what happens in the heart. Aschoff bodies invade all the layers of the heart, where they may produce inflammation of the pericardium, the myocardium, and the endocardium.

The dangerous part is the inflammation of the endocardium. Aschoff bodies form masses in the leaflets of the valves. As they heal, these masses will scar and distort the valve, sticking the edges of the leaflets together with adhesions or pulling the leaflets out of shape so that they leak. Sometimes they do both (Fig. 14-2).

The mitral valve is the one most often affected. When a physician detects mitral stenosis he or she can be sure it's the result of rheumatic fever—there is no other cause. Mitral regurgitation can also be caused by rheumatic fever, but often it is the result of degeneration of the supporting tissues of the valve by a number of other diseases. Aortic stenosis and regurgitation can also be caused by rheumatic carditis (see Chap. 10). Rheumatic fever tends to involve more than one valve; when the aortic valve is diseased, it's almost certain the mitral valve will also be involved to some extent. In severe cases all four valves can be involved.

There are some characteristics of rheumatic heart disease that everyone involved in the care of children and adolescents should know.

1. Rheumatic fever occurs most commonly in the age group 5–15, in the fall, winter, and spring months. In other words, it is primarily a disease of schoolchildren during the school year.

2. The streptococcal sore throat that brings on rheumatic fever is often so mild the child never sees a physician. A physician cannot tell if a sore throat is a strep throat by looking at it.

3. The only way to diagnose a strep throat is by a throat culture.

4. If a strep throat is diagnosed early and treated properly, rheumatic fever will not occur.

5. Proper treatment for a strep throat means 10 days of an adequate level of the right antibiotic in the body—never less. Penicillin is excellent, and the strep never becomes resistant to it. If the patient is allergic to penicillin, other antibiotics can be used. Sulfa drugs should never be used for strep throat; they don't prevent rheumatic fever.

DIAGNOSING RHEUMATIC FEVER IS DIFFICULT

All too often the victim of rheumatic fever has no idea there's anything wrong. In over 50% of cases there won't be any sore joints or skin rashes and the strep throat is passed off as a cold.

With luck, a competent physician may detect the murmur of valvular disease during a routine examination. Otherwise, the disease strikes out of silence. Most of the time it's an insidious process that doesn't make its presence known until the heart is seriously compromised. The first warning the patient may have is the appearance of shortness of breath in early adult life.

A typical example I saw a few years ago was a 28-year-old woman who was 8 months pregnant. The increased workload of pregnancy plus stenosis of the mitral valve pushed her into severe congestive heart failure. The frightening fact was that she had no idea there was anything wrong with her heart until she started gasping for air and coughing blood. In 1938, she would almost certainly have died and the baby with her. In 1988, a heart surgeon opened the valve, and a healthy baby was delivered a month later: a happy outcome.

Rheumatic valvular disease progresses slowly from childhood through adolescence. Symptoms usually appear in early adult life. In the great majority of cases, there is still plenty of time for surgical correction. Sometimes rheumatic valvular disease is so mild the patient has no symptoms at all, while in other slightly more severe cases it can be managed medically through a normal lifetime.

On the basis of the symptoms and the findings of physical examination, a skilled cardiologist can, in a few minutes, diagnose rheumatic valvular disease precisely, including the valve or valves involved, the type of disease (stenosis or regurgitation), and the severity of the disease in terms of load on the heart. By using other diagnostic aids such as an electrocardiogram, an x-ray of the chest, and an echocardiogram, it is possible to be almost mathematically exact. This kind of assessment calls for highly honed medical skills, and patients should never settle for less. When there's a question of evaluating a heart murmur or abnormal heart sounds or possible heart symptoms, get an expert!

THE COURSE OF RHEUMATIC FEVER

Once the rheumatic process has started, there is nothing modern medical science can to do to alter it. The disease is going to run its course and the physician can only watch for signs of cardiac involvement and treat them when possible. Sometimes the acute rheumatic process involves all the layers of the heart—epicardium, myocardium, and endocardium—in what is called "pancarditis." Even today, this can be fatal; steroids and other supportive measures are used, but it's not clear how much they help. (A few years ago, I saw a 10-year-old child come close to dying from rheumatic pancarditis after his parents had refused treatment for two documented streptococcal infections of the throat. He subsequently underwent surgery for aortic valve replacement.)

In the acute stage of rheumatic carditis, various disorders of rhythm and conduction may appear—most commonly, minor degrees of AV nodal block and nodal tachycardias.

The sore joints and other signs of rheumatic inflammation may go on for months. Certain blood tests will remain positive or elevated all this time, specifically, the sedimentation rate and the various antistreptococcal antibodies. Steroids produce a deceptive improvement at this stage. The joints clear up wonderfully, the patient feels just fine, and the sedimentation rate returns to normal. The sad fact, however, is that the lesions in the heart progress inexorably: steroids, in other words, make the patient feel much better *but they do nothing to prevent rheumatic valvular heart disease*.

After an average of 9 months, the rheumatic process will have run its course. If the heart is involved, the abnormality should be detectable by this time.

Practical note: Murmurs indicating mitral valve involvement are often heard during the acute stage; however, it is never certain at this point that there will be significant permanent valvular damage. After the acute attack, what? The physician has two responsibilities at this point.

FIVE COMMANDMENTS FROM ON HIGH ABOUT RHEUMATIC FEVER AND RHEUMATIC HEART DISEASE

1. Rheumatic fever is always caused by infection of the nasopharynx with the group A beta-hemolytic streptococcus.
2. Streptococcal pharyngitis is diagnosed when there is any combination of signs or symptoms of pharyngitis and a positive throat culture.
3. Giving appropriate antibiotic therapy within one week of onset of the streptococcal pharyngitis will prevent rheumatic fever. Rheumatic heart disease is completely preventable; it's the only kind of heart disease that is.
4. Once rheumatic fever starts, it's going to run its course and the physician can only watch and pray that the heart isn't involved.
5. Rheumatic fever is a disease of recurrence. Any patient with documented rheumatic fever should be maintained on secondary prophylaxis indefinitely—certainly well into adult life.

First, if cardiac involvement is present, the physician is committed to continuing careful monitoring to see if the valve damage is severe and if surgery is needed.

Second, the physician must be even more committed to preventing a recurrence. Recurrence of rheumatic fever is common. Once the immune track is "set up," the next attack of streptococcal pharyngitis is very likely to produce another attack with more heart damage. Rheumatic fever is characteristically a disease of recurrence, and in the days before antibiotics, recurrences were the rule. These recurrences are completely preventable.

The group A beta-hemolytic streptococcus never becomes resistant to penicillin. (That's the one good thing about this particular bacillus.) Therefore, anyone who has had documented rheumatic fever should be given adequate doses of penicillin to prevent recurrent streptococcal infections until well into adult life. This can be accomplished by means of monthly injections of benzathine penicillin or twice-daily oral penicillin. With this regime, there is about 98% protection against recurrences. If a patient cannot take penicillin, sulfa drugs or other antibiotics can be used. (Sulfa drugs are worthless for the treatment of streptococcal pharyngitis, but they are excellent for prevention—that is, for keeping the streptococcus out of the body in the first place.) Doctors and nurses must be aware that many laypersons share the following mistaken notion: "Hey, wait a minute! If you give people penicillin for a long time they get resistant to it. It won't do them any good when they need it for something else." Absolutely, 180 degrees wrong. Nobody ever develops resistance to an antibiotic. Some germs do, some don't—but the human body never does. The streptococcus of rheumatic fever never develops resistance to penicillin. A patient could take penicillin for secondary prophylaxis for 20 years, and on 20 years plus 1 day the penicillin would be as effective as ever if a new strep germ turned up. It would be equally effective for pneumonia, or meningitis, or anything else. The effect of the antibiotic depends entirely on the germ—not on the patient.

CHAPTER 15

Pregnancy and Heart Disease

Pregnancy and labor increase the workload on the heart for several reasons. The chief one is that the heart has to pump more blood to meet the extra requirements of the fetus and the tissues that support it. The total volume of blood during a woman's first pregnancy increases by about 40% to 50%. With succeeding pregnancies or with twins, the increase is greater. At the end of the eighth month, the blood volume stabilizes and remains high until after delivery. In other words, in terms of cardiac work, a pregnant woman is walking up a hill for 9 months, with no way to stop.

Pregnancy has other effects on the circulation. The body tends to hold salt and water, so that most pregnant women have obvious edema. In the later stages of pregnancy, the pressure of the fetal sac on the veins of the pelvis and legs often leads to congestion of the veins with risk of clots. A healthy woman can adjust to all these changes with little risk to herself or the baby. Some women with heart disease can go through pregnancy with no real increase in risk, while others face a risk so high that pregnancy should be prevented or terminated.

What kind of heart disease is a pregnant woman likely to have? Certainly she will not have coronary artery disease. With the rarest of exceptions, coronary disease is unknown in menstruating women.

Rheumatic heart disease is now extremely rare, but it does emerge occasionally and must be dealt with. Hypertension is much more common and presents some specific hazards. Myocarditis or myocardiopathy is rare but dangerous. One specific kind of myocardiopathy associated with pregnancy is especially malignant. Congenital heart disease should have been corrected by the time a woman reaches childbearing age, but there are lapses when medical care is inadequate. I have personally seen a woman reach her eighth month of pregnancy before she presented with an obvious ductus arteriosus.

Before discussing specifics, it's necessary to understand the functional classification of heart disease. This system was developed by the New York Heart Association and it has proved remarkably reliable (Fig. 15–1).

Functional Grade I: This group includes patients who have heart disease but can carry out any ordinary and even most heavy activities without symptoms or difficulty. These patients have no limitations on physical activity.

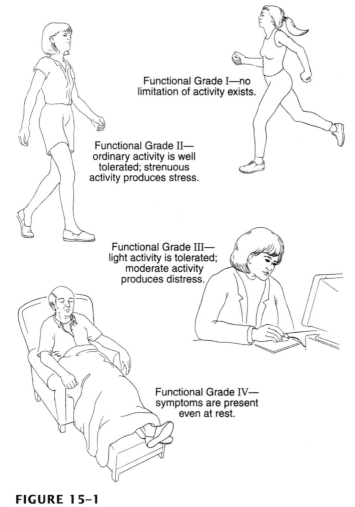

Functional Grade I—no limitation of activity exists.

Functional Grade II—ordinary activity is well tolerated; strenuous activity produces stress.

Functional Grade III—light activity is tolerated; moderate activity produces distress.

Functional Grade IV—symptoms are present even at rest.

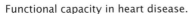

FIGURE 15–1
Functional capacity in heart disease.

Functional Grade II: This includes heart patients who can carry out ordinary physical activity, such as walking, light athletics, and the work of most day-by-day occupations in our society. However, extraordinary exertion such as mountain climbing, strenuous athletics, running, and the like will produce difficulties and must be avoided.

Functional Grade III: This group of patients will suffer symptoms such as shortness of breath or pain even during light-to-moderate activity. A woman carrying bundles from the supermarket to her car, a man walking eight blocks from his home to work, or a golfer strolling about the links would notice some limitation of activity because of these symptoms.

Functional Grade IV: This is the seriously ill group, with symptoms even at rest in a chair or in bed.

Women in functional grade I need have no fear of childbearing. They can produce large families with no more risk than their totally healthy sisters.

Women in functional grade II have much the same outlook, with one important reservation: grade II takes a lot of defining and covers a great many different types of activity. A patient on the borderline between grade II and grade III should approach pregnancy with caution.

Women in functional grade III should not become pregnant. Some of them will be able to carry a child and survive delivery, but a significant proportion will not. All patients in this group can expect to have serious problems in the last 3 months of pregnancy, and there is a good chance that they will go into congestive heart failure during this period, during labor, or during the dangerous 48 hours after delivery.

Women in functional grade IV should never become pregnant. If they do, the pregnancy should be promptly terminated. The chances that the mother will die are very great and the prospects of a normal baby are not very good. The impaired oxygen delivery of a severely failing heart greatly increases chances of miscarriage or fetal deformity.

What are the specific hazards the heart patient faces during pregnancy and labor? A woman in functional grade III or IV is almost certain to go into congestive heart failure during the last 3 months of pregnancy.

The strain of labor throws an additional load on the heart, and many women go into a kind of heart failure that does not respond well to medical management during labor and delivery.

After the placenta has separated from the uterus, the pattern of blood flow in the body changes drastically. For this and other reasons, the first 48 hours after delivery are especially dangerous in women with serious heart disease.

Other hazards of pregnancy such as blood clots in the lung, shock, and hemorrhage are more common and more dangerous in pregnant women with heart disease than in healthy women.

Finally, a rule for physicians and patients alike: **Any woman who has had congestive heart failure before pregnancy is absolutely certain to go into congestive heart failure during her pregnancy despite intensive medical management**.

SPECIAL CONSIDERATIONS

Hypertension

If a woman suffers from mild-to-moderate essential hypertension without complications, she can go through pregnancy without undue risk, provided intensive and competent medical management is available. It is important to control the hypertension, and the physician must realize that some drugs cannot be used because of their effects on the fetus.

Twenty to thirty percent of hypertensive women will develop the condition called preeclampsia, with evidence of abnormal kidney function and danger of convulsions if treatment is not prompt. This danger can be foreseen and prevented, but medical observation must be intense and competent. Severe hypertension, especially if it is not well controlled with drugs, poses a serious risk—the growth of the fetus may be retarded and the risk of maternal death is increased.

Anticoagulants

Many heart conditions require anticoagulant therapy with Coumadin. No woman should ever attempt to go through pregnancy while taking Coumadin. The chances of producing a terribly deformed baby are very high. If a woman is determined to have a child, she can use the injectable form of the anticoagulant heparin throughout pregnancy, administering the medication herself, just as a diabetic takes insulin.

Peripartum Cardiomyopathy

Some years ago at the university hospital, I cared for a woman who was in terminal heart failure from the special kind of degeneration of the heart muscle called peripartum cardiomyopathy. She had 12 children and her heart had failed progressively during the last two pregnancies. There was little we could do except to ease her symptoms. She died of congestive heart failure.

Peripartum cardiomyopathy is a mysterious and dangerous inflammation and degeneration of heart muscle that usually appears in the first 6 months after delivery. In a small percentage of cases the disease appears in late pregnancy, just before birth.

The cause of the disease is unknown. It is thought to be an autoimmune disease like rheumatic fever, with specific antibodies in the mother's blood attacking the heart muscle. The ventricles become dilated and flabby, and congestive heart failure follows quickly. This disease is more common in black women, in women with multiple births, and in older women. In some cases the disease clears remarkably, leaving little aftermath, while in others the heart is damaged permanently. Nobody really knows what causes this disease, and nobody knows how to prevent it. One thing is known beyond question about peripartum cardiomyopathy—any woman who has survived peripartum cardiomyopathy should never become pregnant again.

Rheumatic Carditis

Acute rheumatic carditis with inflammation of all the heart tissues still occurs in Third World countries. It is very dangerous; death during or after labor is common. Pregnancy should practically always be terminated in women with rheumatic carditis.

Labor and delivery can lead to endocarditis. Any woman with valvular or congenital disease should receive endocarditis prophylaxis at the time of delivery and for a suitable period thereafter.

Congenital Heart Defects

Practically all abnormalities of the heart valves can be corrected surgically, and the patient may then be able to go through pregnancy with a good outcome. The point is that all this must be done *before* the heart is damaged beyond recovery. Furthermore, surgery should be performed before pregnancy. It is possible for pregnant women to undergo open-heart surgery, but the ordeal of 3 or more hours on the heart–lung machine is not one the mother or fetus should have to undergo. The risk is high for both.

Congenital heart abnormalities such as patent ductus or coarctation can also be corrected to permit subsequent safe pregnancy and labor.

While there have been some grim passages in this chapter, it ends on a brighter note. Modern medical advances have made it possible to offer a reasonably safe pregnancy and delivery to women who would have been denied childbirth in years past, and the prospect is improving every year.

Notes: *Be sure you understand the New York Heart Association's functional classification system and the relation of each class to risk during pregnancy.*

Any woman with any structural abnormality of the heart, acquired or congenital, must receive endocarditis prophylaxis during and after labor and delivery.

Any woman who has been in congestive heart failure before *pregnancy will absolutely, predictably go into congestive heart failure during pregnancy or delivery.*

If a woman must take Coumadin she cannot carry a pregnancy: the odds are overwhelming that the fetus will be dead or terribly deformed.

No woman who has suffered one episode of peripartum cardiomyopathy should ever become pregnant again.

CHAPTER 16

Pulmonary Heart Disease

This chapter is about the way chronic lung disease affects the cardiovascular system. Many kinds of lung disease create a barrier to the flow of blood from the right heart into the lungs. This happens because of scarring and other changes in the lungs. The high resistance to blood flow causes back pressure in the pulmonary arteries, the right heart, and the veins of the body. This increased pressure forces edema fluid out into the tissues. The condition is called **cor pulmonale,** or pulmonary heart disease.

Chronic lung disease and the pulmonary heart disease that goes with it is one of the most common causes of disability and slow death in the Western world today. It is 90% caused by humans and often totally unnecessary. Remember right heart failure? Look again at Figure 6–5 and reread the section on right heart failure in Chapter 7.

CHRONIC OBSTRUCTIVE PULMONARY DISEASE

Far and away the most common cause of pulmonary heart disease is the condition called chronic obstructive pulmonary disease (COPD). It's a combination of emphysema and bronchitis. It comes in two principal forms. You've seen many victims of this disease in public places and you would certainly have been aware that they were very sick—sometimes in agony. Typically, you would have seen an older person who was fighting for breath in a peculiar way. The victim would inhale with a sudden effort and then force the breath out with a prolonged, audible sigh, often with a wheeze. You would guess that the patient actually had to force the air out of the lungs, and you'd be right. What you were looking at was emphysema.

In this disease, the small air cells of the lungs rupture into large, inefficient sacs. These sacs don't exchange oxygen very well, and they tend to trap air (Fig. 16–1). They act exactly like the Chinese finger trap of your childhood: you could push your finger in, but you couldn't pull it back out.

The trapping of air in these sacs causes the long, slow, agonizing exhalations of emphysema. The patient does manage to get enough oxygen into the body, but it's done with tremendous effort. For that reason, these patients are called **pink puffers.**

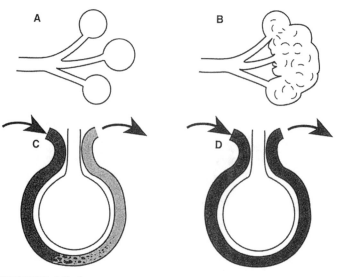

FIGURE 16–1

A. The alveoli are normally separate small sacs, like grapes on the end of stems. **B.** With emphysema, many alveoli rupture, forming large inefficient sacs. **C.** Normally, blood carries oxygen away from the lungs. **D.** When air cells are plugged, blood from the veins flows through the lungs without picking up oxygen.

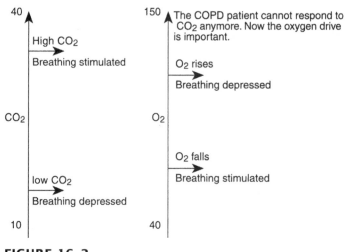

FIGURE 16–2

Regulation of breathing.

Chronic inflammation of the smaller bronchioles, or bronchiolitis, is the other element of COPD. Imagine the worst runny nose you ever had and picture the same process in all the small air passages. This disease has a different effect on the function of the lungs. The inflammation of the bronchioles blocks the passage of air; many alveoli receive little or no air.

Blood passing by these alveoli doesn't pick up any oxygen and goes on into the arterial circulation as dark venous blood (Fig. 16–2). For these reasons, the patient will have a bluish discoloration in addition to being very short of breath. These patients are called **blue bloaters;** they're much sicker than the pink puffers because the oxygen level in their blood is low and the carbon dioxide is high. Remember, no exchange of oxygen or carbon dioxide has taken place in the diseased segments of the lungs, and what's coming out into the arterial vessels is "dirty" venous blood with very little oxygen and a lot of carbon dioxide.

The blue bloaters get in trouble for several reasons. One reason is that the "thermostat" in the brain that regulates breathing is reset, so that breathing is depressed. Thermostat? Some explanation is needed.

THE BREATHING THERMOSTAT AND HOW IT WORKS

The following is important basic information for anyone involved in the care of patients with chronic lung disease.

There are cells in the part of the brain called the brain stem that help to regulate the force of breathing. They respond to changes in the oxygen and carbon dioxide levels in the blood just the way a thermostat responds to changes in the temperature. These cells are called the breathing center.

If a spoiled 5-year-old tells you he's going to hold his breath until he gets his way, tell him to go ahead. After about 30 seconds, he'll gasp for air. He can't control his response. The reason is that while he held his breath, carbon dioxide was piling up rapidly in his blood. When it reaches a certain level, it triggers a reflex through the breathing center. This reflex is so strong he has to breathe. Nobody can hold his breath long enough to hurt himself.

In normal people, the level of carbon dioxide is what regulates breathing. In the blue-bloater group, the carbon dioxide is high all the time, so that the cells of the breathing center become used to this high level. It takes an even higher level to stimulate them. The cells behave like a child who is corrupted by being paid a dollar for a job she used to do for a nickel. There's no way she is going to respond to a nickel anymore. Finally, the cells of the breathing center don't respond to high carbon dioxide levels at all.

Now the patient has to depend on the oxygen level in the blood to drive the breathing center. If the oxygen level falls below a certain point, breathing will be stimulated. This system tends to "wear out" too, so that finally breathing is so depressed that the patient is in danger of dying.

If you give oxygen to someone with a severely depressed breathing center you can kill the patient. The breathing center has been set for a low blood oxygen level. If the oxygen level rises, breathing will stop because the breathing center is turned off. In other words, the rise in oxygen tells the cells in the breathing center they don't need to turn on the breathing reflex anymore.

Since the carbon dioxide level lost its power to stimulate long ago, there's nothing left to drive the breathing center. Death can follow quickly.

Oxygen must be administered at a low level to give the body time to "reset" to new blood oxygen and carbon dioxide levels. The levels of oxygen and carbon dioxide in the blood must be monitored carefully. Too much oxygen can depress breathing and cause the carbon dioxide to rise dangerously. Sometimes it's necessary to insert a breathing tube into the patient's windpipe and use an artificial ventilator.

When the blood oxygen falls or the carbon dioxide rises, the pulmonary arteries will constrict. This constriction is actually caused by the change in the blood gases. With the constriction of the arteries, the pressure in the pulmonary vessels rises. This high pressure backs up into the right heart and out into the veins. The high pressure in the veins forces edema fluid out into the tissues. The liver will enlarge because it's distended with blood and the ankles will swell because of the natural tendency of water to move downhill. In severe cases the abdomen may fill with water (ascites).

This is the whole dismal picture of COPD leading to chronic cor pulmonale. What's even more dismal is that it doesn't need to happen. It's usually a self-inflicted disease. **The majority of all COPD cases occur in heavy smokers.**

Chronic asthma can lead to COPD. So can inhalation of asbestos fibers and silica dust. (Fortunately these two poisons have been largely eliminated from the environment.) Rare diseases like sarcoidosis can lead to COPD. Tuberculosis used to be a common cause of COPD, but it's very rare today. Together, these causes account for only about 5% to 10% of all cases of COPD.

TREATMENT OF COPD

It's relatively easy to pull the edema fluid out of the body through the kidneys with diuretic drugs. The trouble is that the relief is temporary. The cause of the trouble is in the lungs. It's not always possible to do much about the disease in the lungs once it's well established. Some measures can help, especially if the disease isn't too far gone.

Raising the oxygen level in the blood helps in two ways. First, the tissues of the body can begin to function more normally with an adequate supply of oxygen, their vital fuel. Second, the pressure in the blood vessels in the lungs may drop toward normal after the blood oxygen has been near normal for a time. Prolonged use of oxygen, properly administered, has been shown to go far toward alleviating chronic cor pulmonale.

The smaller airways of the lungs can be opened with several types of medication. Infections of the lungs can be treated with appropriate antibiotics. In some cases, modified exercise programs can improve the lungs' ability to function. Intensive treatment of asthma and tuberculosis, especially in the early stages, can prevent the scarring and other changes in the lungs that lead to COPD.

COPD can be stopped and even reversed if it's caught in the early stages. The vital part of treatment is stopping smoking. If the patient goes on smoking, there's little hope of changing the course of the disease.

Of course, the simplest and the most inexpensive approach to COPD is prevention. Lifestyle changes would dramatically lower the incidence of COPD.

CHAPTER 17

Imaginary Heart Disease

SYNDROME X

A 50-year-old woman feels pain behind her breastbone when she walks or cleans house. The pain is pressing, "like someone squeezing her chest." When she stops, the pain goes away. Sometimes the relation to exertion is variable. The woman may notice that even if she goes on exercising the pain goes away. At other times it may appear at rest. She consults a physician who tells her the pain sounds like angina pectoris and orders further tests. The resting electrocardiogram shows some nonspecific abnormalities of the ST–T complex. A treadmill test is strongly positive; the patient feels pain and the ST segment goes down 1.5 mm at a moderate level of exercise. All this looks dangerous, so the physician orders coronary arteriography.

Surprise! The coronary arteriography is completely normal. The left ventricle pumps normally. There's nothing wrong with the heart. If the physician isn't well informed, he will be baffled. If he knows as much as he should, he'll realize the patient is very lucky. She has a syndrome called **Likoff-X** in honor of Dr. William Likoff, who did many of the early studies on it. It's a medical curiosity, but it's not a disease.

Nobody has any idea why menopausal and postmenopausal women have this pseudoangina syndrome. A great deal of research has failed to reveal the cause. Some studies have suggested that there is some abnormality in the circulation through the small vessels or capillaries of the heart muscle, but there's no agreement on what it is or even if it exists.

One thing is absolutely clear, however—it's harmless. The woman with syndrome X can take up mountain climbing or weight lifting or singles tennis or whatever suits her fancy. In spite of the abnormal ECG and stress test, the woman has a normal life expectancy and has no reason to fear heart trouble. Syndrome X does not produce any bad effects and there is no risk of disease or death. It's not a disease by any reasonable definition. It's an oddity; no more serious than having one blue eye and one brown one. The intelligent physician explains all this to the woman and gives her something like aspirin for the pain in her chest.

Physicians sometimes prescribe cardiac medications in an unthinking reflex response to the pain in the chest and the abnormal ECG. This is a bad idea for several reasons. In the first place, the cardiac medications don't do any good because there's nothing to treat. In the second place, the mere act of taking cardiac medications often makes the patient a "cardiac cripple." She becomes convinced that there must be something the matter with her heart when, in fact, there isn't. Furthermore, medications are often toxic.

IMAGINARY SPASM

The coronary arteries can squeeze shut, even when there's no actual disease. Spasm of an anatomically normal coronary artery can produce angina pectoris. In rare cases it can even cause myocardial infarction. Spasm of coronary arteries often produces the characteristic pattern of Prinzmetal angina, described in Chapter 8. The ECG will show elevation of the ST segment during pain, with prompt return to normal when the pain stops. The best way to diagnose coronary spasm is to detect the ECG changes during pain by means of a Holter monitor recording. With the newer models, ST deviation can be precisely recorded; the combination of symptoms and ECG change establishes the diagnosis.

There are a couple of ways to bring on coronary spasm artificially. One is hyperventilation. The patient is instructed to breathe deeply, rapidly, and regularly for at least 30 seconds. For some reason, this can cause a sensitive coronary artery to go into spasm. This will only happen, it should be noted, if the artery already has a tendency to spasm. Spasm can also be produced by injecting a drug called ergonovine directly into a coronary artery. This is a stronger stimulus, but it's not totally safe. Ergonovine is so potent that sometimes the spasm it produces doesn't relax and the patient can suffer a myocardial infarct. There was a wave of enthusiasm for the use of ergonovine to detect spasm about 10 years ago, and the cardiology journals were awash with articles about coronary spasm. Now you rarely hear about the subject. (Medical science tends to go in vogues and trends.)

The enthusiasm for spasm had one really bad aftermath. Thoughtless physicians all too often use the term *spasm* to excuse their failure to find a cause of chest pain. A patient, typically female, presents with chest pain that might or might not be anginal. All tests are negative, but instead of sending the patient on her way with reassurance and advice to live a normal life, the less than competent physician will tell the patient that she "probably has coronary spasm." He then prescribes assorted cardiac medication, constricts the patient's life, destroys her insurability, and probably makes her a nervous wreck. This is brainless and cannot be condoned and is like telling someone they "might have a little cancer," or possibly "might be a little pregnant." It should never be done without hard-core evidence that spasm is in fact present. True, isolated coronary spasm in otherwise normal coronary arteries is a rare condition that deserves very careful study to substantiate the diagnosis. To say that a patient has coronary spasm on the basis of vague chest pain without one or more of the types of objective evidence listed above is inexcusable and falls below any acceptable standard of practice.

CASUAL CORONARY ARTERY DISEASE

A patient describes chest pain that may or may not be suggestive of coronary disease. The physician tells the patient to take nitroglycerin or beta blockers or calcium blockers because the patient "might have coronary disease." To tell a patient that he or she "might" have a major disease without moving heaven and earth to establish the diagnosis is worse than medical incompetence. It falls below the level of ordinary common sense.

Before a patient is saddled with a diagnosis of coronary artery disease, the physician should be sure beyond reasonable doubt that the disease is really present. The ECG, the stress test, the isotope test, and the coronary arteriogram are all available, and there's no excuse for not making a precise diagnosis. The implications of coronary artery disease are so profound in terms of medical management, lifestyle, insurability, occupation, and family plans that the physician is justified in going to any reasonable lengths to clarify the diagnosis.

CHAPTER 18

To Pace or Not to Pace

Cardiac pacemakers represent one of the great accomplishments of 20th-century cardiology. Before pacemakers were available, there was no treatment for diseases that produced a slow heart rate—or no rate at all. Patients became dizzy, or fainted, or died when failure of the sinoatrial node or the AV conducting system dropped the heart rate below a level that could sustain health or life. Until the 1960s, physicians could only watch helplessly and prescribe drugs that had little effect. Then came pacemakers.

A cardiac pacemaker is simply an electrode attached at one end to the heart and at the other to an electric power pack that sends out an impulse very like the normal activating wave that makes the heart beat. The speed and intensity of the impulse can be controlled and a suitable heart rhythm can be restored.

Modern pacemakers are a triumph of engineering. With one electrode in the atria and one in the ventricle, a pacemaker can make the heart beat in a normal, synchronized manner. It can sense changes in hemodynamics and adjust itself to the needs of the patient. A pacemaker has safety features that permit it to recognize the patient's own heartbeat and change accordingly. There are many different types of pacemakers to suit almost any clinical setting.

There are still technical problems—lead wires can break and power units can malfunction—but, on balance, the evolution of modern pacemakers has been a marvel of engineering.

On the medical side, things have sometimes been less than marvelous. There's been confusion about the indications for permanent pacing, and it seems clear that a significant number of patients have received pacemakers who didn't need them. Those of us who train physicians to interpret electrocardiograms have been deeply concerned about the failure of many cardiology training programs in recent years to teach this subject adequately. Experts in the field are lamentably sparse—a condition some of us are trying to correct. There really shouldn't be any doubt about the indications for permanent pacing. They've been obvious for many years to every physician who has worked in the field of the arrhythmias. For all these reasons, the indications for implantation of a permanent pacemaker are spelled out here as plainly and simply as possible.

Important Note: Implantation of a permanent pacemaker is never an emergency. A temporary pacing wire can be floated into the heart easily and safely and can be kept there long enough to permit careful clinical evaluation and expert consultation. That pacemaker may be going in for a lifetime, and it's not innocuous. Any patient deserves a couple of opinions and long, careful consideration before a pacemaker is implanted.

HOW TO TELL WHEN SOMEONE NEEDS A PACEMAKER

I had the privilege of serving as chairman of a committee of distinguished cardiologists who published guidelines for pacing in the *Journal of the American Medical Association*.[1] It's possible to condense these guidelines as follows:

Complete Heart Block in the Bundle Branch System

If nothing can travel from the atria to the ventricles because both bundle branches are permanently out of action and can't conduct, permanent pacing is always indicated.

Mobitz Type II Block

Properly diagnosed, this means that one bundle branch is permanently blocked and the other fails now and then. The risk of catastrophe in these patients is over 30% per year. Permanent pacing is justified whether or not the patient has symptoms. Remember, Mobitz II block happens only in the setting of preexisting bundle branch block. Thus the QRS will be wide. If a physician makes a diagnosis of Mobitz II block when the QRS is narrow, the patient should run, not walk, to another, more competent physician. A narrow QRS means that both bundle branches are functioning normally. Mobitz II block in the presence of a narrow QRS is one of the rarest phenomena in electrocardiography.

Intrinsic, Permanent, or Severely Recurrent AV Nodal Block—High Degree or Complete (Rare)

This must be distinguished from insignificant AV nodal block. It's not unusual for healthy people to have short periods of block in the AV node. Studies in Israel and Britain have documented Wenckebach and first-degree AV nodal block in healthy young people, especially at night. It's a normal variant. Remember that the vagus nerve goes to the AV node and stimulation of the vagus nerve can produce transient AV nodal block. Retching and vomiting are common causes of vagal stimulation. Many normal people reading this have certainly had periods of AV nodal block during the peak of a hangover or while reacting to spoiled potato salad. Many drugs depress conduction through the AV node, such as digitalis, calcium blockers, and beta blockers, which all can produce AV nodal block alone. Add the vagal effect of retching and the block can be dramatic. Morphine, Demerol, and related pain-killing drugs stimulate the vagus powerfully. I have seen cases when pacemakers were implanted on the basis of periods of AV nodal block obviously produced by drugs, by the vagal stimulation of nausea and vomiting, or by both, sometimes with tragic results.

If AV nodal block appears during periods of intense vagal stimulation or drug effect, a temporary pacing wire can be inserted. The honest, competent physician will then wait for these temporary effects to wear off before recommending a permanent pacemaker. Ninety-nine times out of a hundred, the AV block will disappear. The word *intrinsic* in the earlier heading means that there's something wrong with the cells of the AV node itself. To justify pacing, the block must either be permanent or must recur often enough to be a hazard. The word *permanent* is especially important when a patient suffers an infarct involving the right coronary artery. This artery supplies the AV node most of the time. Temporary AV nodal block is common during an inferior myocardial infarct. Temporary pacing may be needed. Permanent pacing is never needed: the AV node always recovers. It may take up to 2 weeks, but the AV node will come back to normal.

Now the words at the beginning of this heading should take on specific meaning. True, intrinsic, permanent, or severely recurrent high-degree or complete AV nodal block is rare.

Warning for patients and referring physicians: If AV block is present and if the QRS is narrow, the block must be in the AV node. The chances are then overwhelming that the block is caused by drugs or by some temporary effect such as ischemia or vagal effect. Don't let anyone implant a permanent pacemaker until all these possibilities have been thoroughly excluded.

Sick Sinus Syndrome

Most permanent pacemaker insertions are for the sick sinus syndrome. True sick sinus syndrome is rare. Abnormally slow sinus rates are usually caused by drugs. The list of drugs that depress the sinus node is remarkable. It includes digitalis, quinidine, calcium blockers, beta blockers, clonidine, amiodarone, and drugs used for agitated psychic states, among others. Infarction involving the right coronary artery often produces a temporary slow sinus rate. If all these outside influences have been excluded, and if a slow sinus rate causes symptoms, the sick sinus syndrome is present and a permanent pacemaker is needed.

What symptoms? Dizziness and fainting. The patient may feel close to fainting without actually losing consciousness (presyncope). These are the only true symptoms of the sick sinus syndrome. Very rarely, a slow heart rate may make congestive failure worse. A severely depressed left ventricle may not be able to pump enough blood at a slow rate. The symptoms will then be dyspnea and orthopnea. There's another form of the sick sinus syndrome where bursts of rapid abnormal atrial rhythm alternate with a sinus rate that's slow enough to produce symptoms. The rapid rate may be caused by fibrillation, flutter, or supraventricular tachycardia.

Important distinction: Any of these arrhythmias can occur in short bursts. If the sinus node functions normally between the episodes of rapid beating, the sick sinus syndrome is not present and pacing is not required. If the sinus rate between episodes of tachycardia is so low that it produces symptoms, the bradycardia-tachycardia type of the sick sinus syndrome is present and pacing is indicated.

SPECIAL CASES FOR PERMANENT PACING

Atrial Fibrillation with AV Block

When the atria fibrillate, they bombard the AV node with stimulating impulses about 425 times per minute. If the AV conducting system is healthy, the heart will beat rapidly—often too rapidly. If the heart rate is very slow when the atria are fibrillating, it means that there is AV block. If the rate is slow enough to produce symptoms, and if drug effect has been thoroughly ruled out, pacing is justified. There are no P waves from which to measure, so the presence of block must be deduced from the slow rate.

(I continue to see patients in their seventies and eighties who have chronic atrial fibrillation and a dangerously slow heart rate. The slow heart rate is caused by toxic doses of digoxin, but some physician used this as an excuse to implant a pacemaker.)

Syncope Without Obvious Cause

If the ECG is normal at rest and with exercise, it is most unlikely that heart block or sick sinus are the cause or that pacing will help. Recordings with an event recorder—a device like the Holter monitor—are the best approach in this group. The patient wears a recording ECG that can be activated by the patient or family when symptoms appear. It has a memory loop so that it recalls the ECG for 5 seconds before the recording button is pushed. If the ECG is normal during the syncope, there is no possibility that a pacemaker will help.

Carotid Sinus Syncope

There's a bundle of nerve tissue high up under the jaw, in the fork of the carotid artery, called the carotid body. Massaging or pressing on this nest of nerve cells can stimulate the vagus nerve; this then slows the heart rate by depressing the sinus node or producing AV nodal block. Very rarely, this bit of nerve tissue can become overactive and cause syncope by slowing the heart rate. Patients with an oversensitive carotid sinus may faint any time they touch that area of the neck when shaving or dressing.

Firm pressure on the carotid sinus will produce slowing of the heart in many normal patients. There is no correlation between pauses produced by artificial pressure on the carotid sinus and clinical carotid sinus syncope. Age, diabetes, coronary artery disease, and beta-blocking drugs will all exaggerate the effect of carotid sinus stimulation. Pauses of up to 10 seconds have been reported in patients who have never had any symptoms.

Carotid sinus syncope can be diagnosed only when the normal activity of the patient stimulates the carotid sinus to slow the heart rate or drop the blood pressure in a way that produces symptoms. If slowing of the heart rate is the problem, a pacemaker will help.

One more time: Diagnosis of the type of carotid sinus syncope that can be helped by pacing is based on a slowing of the heart rate during ordinary living activities. The Holter monitor or the event recorder is the ideal tool to make the diagnosis. **True carotid sinus syncope is rare**. I have seen two cases in 50 years.

ADVICE: REFERRING A PATIENT FOR POSSIBLE PACING

- **Always** rule out the effect of drugs as a cause of the slow rate.
- **Always** insist the abnormal slow rate be proved to be permanent or severely recurrent rather than a temporary episode.
- **Question** the diagnosis of "chronotropic incompetence" or "concealed AV block" regarding pacing. These are both imaginary entities. Chronotropic incompetence is supposed to be present when the sinus node doesn't speed up appropriately with exercise. The cardiologist who first described it isn't sure it's an entity at all, and there's no evidence that it justifies pacing.[2] "Concealed AV block" is another figment. If AV block is present it will appear on the surface ECG at rest or during exercise. It's possible to produce AV block artificially in normal people by driving the heart with a pacing wire in the atrium, but this has no correlation with heart block in real life.

- **Question** the use of His bundle recordings or other invasions of the heart with catheters. Many careful studies have shown that all the necessary information about heart block can be learned from the ordinary electrocardiogram. Recordings from within the heart do not add any useful information.
- **Do not** hurry into permanent pacing. There's always time to insert a temporary pacer and get consultation. ECGs can be faxed to anyplace in the country for expert analysis.

TRICUSPID INSUFFICIENCY

Any pacing wire will lie right across the leaflets of the tricuspid valve. These valve leaflets are flaps of thin, living tissue: the mechanical distortion and irritation of the pacing wire can affect them. The leaflet tissue may be distorted and scarred and can contract to such a degree that tricuspid insufficiency may follow. I have seen several of these cases, and a number have been reported in the medical literature. This isn't a life-threatening complication, but insufficiency or "leaking" of the tricuspid valve can lead to serious back-pressure in the veins of the body, with swelling of the feet and ankles, just as in the edema of congestive heart failure. Treatment with diuretic agents will take care of this minor complication.

COMPLICATIONS OF PACEMAKERS

The patient is safely past all these hurdles, and a pacemaker that is really needed is implanted. Any problems? Any complications to be expected? Unfortunately, yes. The patient will find it impossible to obtain life or health insurance (except as a member of some very large group). The patient must avoid various power sources and will be barred from some types of employment. Certain diagnostic modes like magnetic resonance imaging cannot be used. There will be medical complications in a significant number of cases.[3]

Infection

The same Dr. Seymour Furman who invented transvenous pacing reported on over 140 cases with "entrapped" pacemaker leads (electrodes that have permanently grown into the tissue of the heart; over half will do this). Eight percent of these became infected. Some of these infections responded to treatment with antibiotics, but some did not. When they didn't, the lead had to be removed surgically. There was one death with this procedure.[3]

Other investigators have reported risk ranging from 1% to 5% of infection and endocarditis around pacemaker wires. An infected wire usually has to be removed or the infection can't be cleared up. This used to involve open heart surgery with substantial risk. Now, a physician in Miami has perfected a method of removing entrapped leads with a special catheter that is much safer.

Blood Clots

Blood has a tendency to clot around any foreign body inside the heart. I have cared for one case of superior vena cava obstruction when clots around a pacemaker wire blocked the veins draining the head and neck and left a patient's face permanently bloated. I have cared for three other cases where the veins of the upper arm were obstructed by clots that formed around pacing wires; in each case, the whole arm became grotesquely swollen. Reports from around the world indicate that clotting complications can be expected in 1% to 5% of all cases. Clots may form around the pacing wire and send emboli, or small bits of clots, into the blood vessels of the lung. It is not known how often this happens.

Mechanical Problems

Broken or malfunctioning lead wires may necessitate removal and repeated surgery.

For the patient who really needs a pacemaker, these complications are insignificant compared to the benefit of a normal heart rhythm. For the patient who doesn't need one, they are tragic.

Something New: Normalizing Pacemakers

A remarkable use of pacemakers has emerged in the last few years. They're used to produce a more powerful, normal contraction when the ventricles aren't synchronized properly. When would that be?

Go back to Chapter 5 and look at the diagrams of the electric system of the heart. Notice that there are two "bundle branches" starting at the AV node and branching down through the ventricles. These are like conducting wires: they carry the activating electric wave down the septum and into the muscle of the two ventricles. Normally they transmit together, at the same speed, so that each ventricle discharges its load of blood at the same instant.

If one of those two bundle branches functions slowly or not at all, the condition is called "bundle branch block." It takes one ventricle longer to be activated than the other, and when they contract, one chamber is ahead of the other. The ventricles contract with an eccentric, uncoordinated motion so the expulsion of blood isn't as smooth and powerful as if the chambers were properly synchronized.

That uncoordinated motion can cut down the efficiency of the heart and if the muscle is otherwise diseased that loss of pumping efficiency may be just enough to put the patient into heart failure.

Since the left ventricle is the powerful pumping ventricle, left bundle branch block was the first condition studied and there appears to be no question that in individuals with depressed cardiac function, this "normalizing" pacemaker in the setting of left bundle branch block can improve cardiac output, relieve symptoms, and *possibly* prolong life—although there are no data yet to prove this.

Other types of conduction delays in the ventricular network are being studied in many centers, always with the hope of improving cardiac performance. The final word is still a good way off.

NOTES

1. Phibbs B, Friedman H, Graboys T, et al. Indications for pacing in the treatment of bradyarrhythmias. *JAMA.* 1984;252:1307–1311.

2. Phibbs B, Marriott HJC. Complications of permanent transvenous pacing. *New Engl J Med.* 1985;312:1428–1432.

3. Furman S. Proceedings, 30th annual scientific session, American College of Cardiology, New Orleans, La. March 18–22, 1990.

CHAPTER 19

Medical Treatment of Heart Failure

This chapter is included here for a good reason. By now the reader should understand what happens when the pumping action of the heart fails. The difference between left heart failure and right heart failure should be clear. The diseases that produce heart failure have been listed and described—hypertension, coronary artery disease, valvular heart disease, disease of the heart muscle, congenital heart disease, chronic lung disease. Now it's time to answer the next question: "What do we do about it?"

Logical answer: "Treat the cause. Remove the cause and prevent the heart failure." Logical answer . . . to a point. Removal of the cause is possible some of the time, but not always. We can control hypertension, we can offset some of the effects of coronary artery disease on heart muscle, we can put in artificial valves or reconstruct some diseased ones, we can repair most types of congenital heart disease. That still leaves some conditions we can't prevent. There are other conditions that could be prevented but often aren't—for instance, hypertensive heart disease when there's poor management or poor cooperation by a patient.

There's really no way of completely preventing coronary artery disease. Even though we can lower the risk, many people are going to lose a critical mass of their left ventricle each year as a result of coronary artery disease. They'll go into congestive failure.

Nobody knows how to prevent myocarditis or myocardiopathy. In most cases, nobody has any idea of the cause.

Sometimes diseased valves aren't detected in time and the heart degenerates past the point of no return.

As long as people pursue activities that are injurious to the heart and lungs, cor pulmonale is going to cripple and kill thousands. In other words, we have to expect heart failure and be ready to treat it.

There are four types of heart failure. It may sound complicated, but the types are usually easy to recognize and differentiate.

ACUTE LEFT HEART FAILURE

There's too much blood in the lungs. It has piled up in the lungs fairly rapidly because the left ventricle isn't pumping the blood out of the lungs as fast as the right ventricle is pumping it in. The lungs are congested with watery fluid and the patient can't get enough oxygen into the blood. The extra fluid may pile up in the tissue spaces around the air passages, or it may actually fill the alveoli (pulmonary edema).

Treatment

Rotating Tourniquets

There's a quick, safe treatment for acute left heart failure that's simple and absolutely free. It doesn't involve pills or shots and no drug company is pushing it for profit. Naturally, the medical profession ignores it.

Remember, the lungs are clogged with fluid so the first thing you want to do is cut down the volume of blood returning to the lungs. Here's a way to do that, but . . . *it's so simple that whole generations of physicians have forgotten it!*

The quickest, safest way to cut down the volume of blood returning to the lungs is to put tourniquets on all four extremities, as high up as possible, and tighten them enough to cut off the veins. Now the blood flows *out* through the arteries, but a great deal of it is trapped in the large reservoirs of veins in the limbs and can't flow *back* to the lungs (Fig. 19–1).

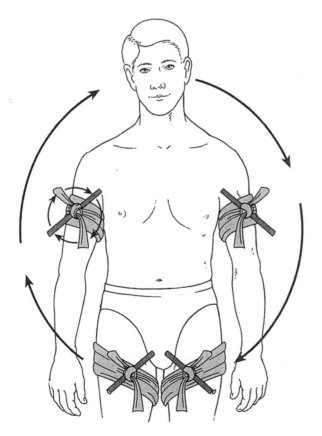

FIGURE 19–1
Rotating tourniquets.

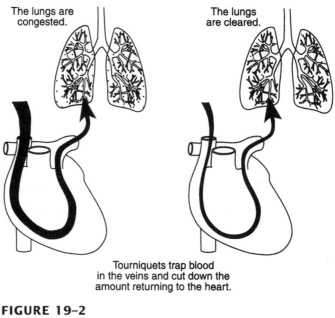

The lungs are congested.

The lungs are cleared.

Tourniquets trap blood in the veins and cut down the amount returning to the heart.

FIGURE 19–2
Congestive heart failure.

With each beat of the heart, the left ventricle is now clearing the lungs of the excess blood (Fig. 19–2). Within a few minutes, the patient will be out of immediate danger. After 15 minutes, one tourniquet is loosened. For as long as needed the tourniquets are rotated—that is, one is loosened every 15 minutes while the other three remain tight.

There is no danger to the circulation in the arms and legs since the arteries aren't turned off. Tourniquets should be available in every coronary intensive care unit in every emergency room, and they should be used freely. They are the safest and best first line of treatment of acute congestive heart failure. (See my comments under "Notes for Critical Care Personnel" at the end of this chapter.)

Diuretics

Furosemide is given by vein. This starts the excess water out through the kidneys (Fig. 19–3). It also drops the pressure in the left atrium. The fall in pressure takes place even before the water starts to leave the body—a bonus effect.

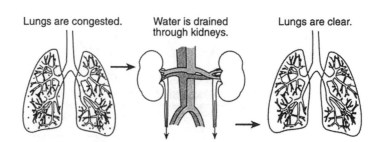

Lungs are congested.

Water is drained through kidneys.

Lungs are clear.

FIGURE 19–3
The effect of diuretics on congested lungs.

Morphine

Morphine dilates the veins and thus has some of the effect of rotating tourniquets. It also helps to turn off some abnormal breathing reflexes, calm the patient, and restore deep, efficient breathing.

Oxygen

As mentioned, the basic problem of acute left heart failure is that oxygen isn't getting from the air into the bloodstream because of the watery congestion in the lungs. Part of the solution, of course, is to give the patient oxygen by mask or nasal cannula.

Therefore the first line of defense is tourniquets, furosemide, morphine, and oxygen (T-F-M-O). Use them all, fast. In the old days, when doctors made housecalls, I would often be summoned to see a patient almost dead of pulmonary edema. I always applied tourniquets and gave morphine. By the time the ambulance arrived, most patients were breathing easily, relaxed, and out of danger.

Instead of applying rotating tourniquets, you can accomplish the same effect by withdrawing 500 cc of blood.

Important Note: If the left heart failure is caused by hypertension, treat the hypertension promptly with nitroprusside. This is a case where a specific cause can be promptly removed.

Digitalis

For generations, physicians have used digitalis in acute left heart failure with the hope that the drug would strengthen the heart muscle. It does have some effect on heart muscle, but it's not very potent. Now that it's possible to measure the performance of the heart very accurately, it has become clear that digitalis has a mildly helpful effect on the pumping action of the heart muscle in acute failure. It's worth using in some cases, but it's not a critical, lifesaving resource as physicians used to think.

Special Warning

The first episode of left heart failure is the most dangerous (Fig. 19–4). The tissue barrier between the blood vessels and the air spaces is thin and easily penetrated. There's very little to keep the fluid in the blood vessels from oozing directly into the alveoli,

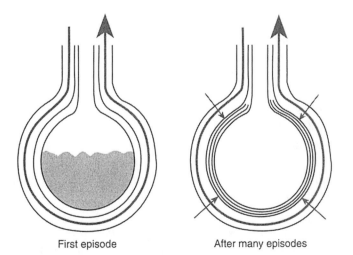

First episode   After many episodes

FIGURE 19–4
Acute left heart failure.

and the lungs fill up fast. After a number of episodes, the tissues in the lungs build up a kind of protective barrier so that it's more difficult for water to ooze from the small pulmonary vessels into the alveoli. In other words, after repeated episodes of congestive heart failure, the lungs tolerate a much higher pressure in the pulmonary capillaries.

Note: The first episode of acute left heart failure may be the last if it's not treated promptly and adequately.

CHRONIC LEFT HEART FAILURE

Some statements are true about any patient with chronic left heart failure. The patient is always **hypervolemic**—in other words, the circulating blood volume is too high. There's excess fluid in the body. In addition, the left ventricle is failing in its job of pumping the blood out of the lungs and on to the body.

To treat left heart failure, it is essential to balance the amount of blood returning to the heart with the amount leaving it. It is also necessary to ensure that there is an adequate flow of well-oxygenated blood leaving the left ventricle to meet the needs of the body.

There are two ways to cut down the amount of blood returning to the heart. The first is diuresis—removing the excess fluid through the kidneys. The second is dilation of the veins with drugs like isosorbide or nitroglycerin. The veins of the body have enormous reserve storage capacity. It is possible to hold a significant amount of blood out in the body and away from the heart by dilating the veins.

These two measures together cut down the volume and pressure of blood returning to the left ventricle. In other words, they cut down on **preload**. At the same time, the volume of blood coming out of the left ventricle can be increased by lowering the resistance in the arteries. This lower resistance means that the ventricle doesn't have to work as hard to pump blood out to the body. The impedance, or resistance, to forward flow in the arteries is called **afterload**. Chronic left heart failure is treated in part by lowering afterload.

Treatment

Diuretics

A whole battery of diuretic drugs now exists, including furosemide, chlorothiazide, bumetanide, and spironolactone, among others.

Giving diuretics without restricting sodium is like mopping up the floor without turning off the leaky faucet. The effect of one heavy overdose of salt can be lethal. Here in Arizona, we often see our Hispanic patients in critical congestive failure because of a liberal serving of *menudo*—a tasty, salt-laden soup—or some other salt-saturated item in the all-too-tempting local cuisine. Be sure you know all about the effect of the diuretic drug on the mineral balance of the body. Dangerous loss of potassium is common; sodium can also fall below the critical level. Different agents have different effects. The health care professional must check on the specific effects of any agent being used.

Spironolactone was originally developed as a diuretic, which it is, but by its action on neutralizing the adrenal secretion called "aldactone" it has proved enormously effective in treatment of congestive heart failure. Unlike some other diuretics, spironolactone causes retention of potassium: it is very important to be aware of this effect.

Lowering Preload

A number of agents can dilate the veins, thereby lowering the load of blood returning to the heart. Nitroglycerin is effective either sublingually or intravenously. Isosorbide has a more prolonged effect when given orally. The problem with the nitrates is they lose their effectiveness very quickly (tachyphylaxis). The veins stop reacting to them in a short time. Recent studies show that the effect of 10 mg of isosorbide taken by mouth is gone in 2 hours after a first dose and in a shorter time than that after succeeding doses. The effect of intravenous nitroglycerin also wears off within a few hours. One way to avoid this loss of effect is to space out the doses or to stop the medication for a time and then renew it.

Nitroprusside dilates both arteries and veins. The effect does not wear off. If the blood pressure doesn't fall too much, it is an excellent drug for acute left heart failure. (However, since nitroprusside can only be given by vein, it can't be used in chronic failure.)

Lowering Afterload

Anything that drops the arterial pressure reduces the afterload. Hydralazine and ACE inhibitors are both effective.

The combination of isosorbide and hydralazine was the first regime shown to be effective in improving cardiac performance in chronic left heart failure. It's safe to say that any patient with congestive heart failure should be given an ACE inhibitor if it's tolerated. (Ace inhibitors make some people cough intolerably: in these the angiotensin-receptor blockers (ARBs) can be given with the same effect and less tendency to produce coughing.)

BETA BLOCKERS

It seems paradoxical, but beta blockers are so useful in congestive heart failure that they should always be employed if possible. The Swedes pioneered the use of beta blockers in this setting: they began with minute doses in the range of 4 mg of propranolol and increased the dose cautiously to the usual daily level. Beta blockers, we now know, produce a slower, more efficient heartbeat. They also block the abnormal catecholamine response of the sympathetic nervous system which can constrict coronary and other arteries. The agents should always be started at low doses and increased with careful observation for untoward effects. They cannot be used if bronchospastic asthma or significant peripheral vascular disease are present.

Carvedilol is a combination of sympathetic blockers that has both alpha and beta effects. In other words, there is some vasodilatation as well as some beta blockade and the combination appears to work well. Whether it is better than the long-acting beta blocker topranolol-xl is still a matter of investigation.

Oxygen

When blood levels are borderline or low, chronic use of low levels of oxygen is sometimes lifesaving. (The Medicare standards that authorize chronic use of oxygen are too stringent. They ignore a large body of work showing that oxygen is very helpful in chronic failure even when blood levels of oxygen are only moderately depressed.) Oxygen should always be part of the treatment of chronic left heart failure.

Digitalis

This familiar drug comes last because it's the least important. Digitalis does have some mild effect in improving cardiac performance in chronic left heart failure, but it's much less than generations of physicians had hoped. Some recent studies have suggested that relatively low levels of digitalis are helpful in chronic heart failure. It is suggested that higher levels that are still within the therapeutic range may be harmful. (I personally doubt this observation very much. Having employed digitalis in thousands of cases, for longer periods than most physicians alive today, I am convinced that the supposed negative effects of this agent are grossly exaggerated.) Some recent studies suggest that digitalis and ACE inhibitors together may be better than either alone. Digitalis is a superb drug for treatment of many arrhythmias, even though its usefulness in heart failure is marginal. (I treat many older patients for the toxic effects of digitalis compounds they didn't need. It's usually given with some vague hope of "strengthening the heart," but all too often it threatens the patient's life.)

ISOLATED OR "PURE" RIGHT HEART FAILURE

This term refers to diseases that affect only the right heart. The two commonest examples are severe chronic pulmonary disease and stenosis of the pulmonic valve. The one manifestation of right heart failure is edema. The treatment is diuresis. When pulmonary artery pressure is elevated as a result of chronic, low blood oxygen, as in COPD, prolonged low levels of oxygen can actually produce permanent lowering of the abnormal pressure, thus improving the right heart failure.

COMBINED HEART FAILURE

The commonest cause of right heart failure is left heart failure. When the left ventricle fails, the pressure backs up through the lungs and into the pulmonary artery and right heart. The patient who presents with dyspnea and edema represents failure of both sides of the heart. The same principles of treatment apply—diuresis, balancing of preload and afterload, and oxygen.

NOTES FOR CRITICAL CARE PERSONNEL

In medical science someone is always rediscovering the wheel. Use of rotating tourniquets in acute heart failure is the best example. Physicians are so conditioned to think of shots and pills that they tend to dismiss simple measures and all too often younger physicians aren't trained in them. Every few years, a paper appears in the leading cardiology journals reporting the marvelous effectiveness and safety of rotating tourniquets for heart failure. The authors always sound surprised. (Older physicians have a hard time keeping a straight face when they read such reports.)

With another turn of the wheel, the most advanced centers have now "rediscovered" tourniquets as the quickest and safest treatment. It is safe to say that any emergency room, paramedic unit, or intensive care unit should be equipped with tourniquets, and personnel should be trained in their use. Tourniquets can be applied anywhere, in any setting, and if used properly are completely safe. They are more effective than intravenous furosemide, oxygen, or, indeed, any other emergency measure.

Note: *Always check to make sure you haven't shut off the arterial pulse. Remember, it doesn't take much pressure to shut off the veins.*

Use your eyes and your watch when you think the patient is in congestive heart failure. Some simple diagnostic observations are universal.

1. The patient in congestive heart failure will always be breathing rapidly. Count the respiratory rate.

2. The breathing will always be shallow. Remember, the lungs are full of water. Continued rapid, *deep* breathing means acidosis—for example, diabetic acidosis. Occasional deep breaths accompanied by panic means hyperventilation—nerves!

3. Unless the patient has heart block or sick sinus syndrome, the heart will always be beating rapidly. Count the pulse.

4. Patients with severe heart failure will almost always be orthopneic—you can't make them lie down, and don't try.

5. Morphine may be lifesaving in acute left heart failure, but it's very dangerous in acute respiratory failure and can kill the patient; so can all the other narcotic agents. The distinction between these two clinical conditions isn't always easy, and critical care personnel should never be put in the position of trying to make this distinction. Even a modest dose of a tranquilizing drug or a hypnotic agent can be lethal. If there's any question, watch for depression of breathing whenever these agents are administered and move quickly if trouble appears.

Remember that water runs downhill. This includes the fluid of cardiac edema. Any patient in congestive heart failure should have the head higher than the feet. A high tilt in bed or an actual reclining chair position keeps the maximum fluid down in the lower extremities and away from the heart. The simple act of moving from sitting or standing to the supine position increases venous return to the heart by at least 30%—enough to give some patients real trouble. Our medical tradition of putting all sick people flat in bed isn't very sensible; when congestive heart failure is present it's downright dangerous.

One more time: Water flows to the lowest point. When swelling in the ankles disappears after the patient is put in bed, don't assume the water's gone. It will move to the lowest point, which will be the area just above the buttocks, around the sacrum. Check for pitting edema there.

CHAPTER 20

Catheterization of the Heart and Coronary Arteriography

A catheter is simply a long, thin, hollow tube of any kind. It's possible to thread a catheter up a vein or an artery and into the heart. If a catheter is threaded up a vein it will move through the inferior or superior vena cava, and then into the right atrium, the right ventricle, and, if desired, into the pulmonary artery (Fig. 20–1).

If it is threaded up an artery it ends up in the left ventricle. It's not practical to try to force a catheter backward across the mitral valve, so the left ventricle is as far as the catheter can go (Fig. 20–2).

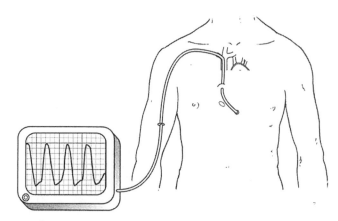

FIGURE 20–1
Catheterization of the right heart. A catheter is threaded up a vein in the arm, through the right atrium, and on into the right ventricle and pulmonary artery. It's possible to measure pressures and oxygen levels at each level; for special tests, dye or radioisotopes can be injected.

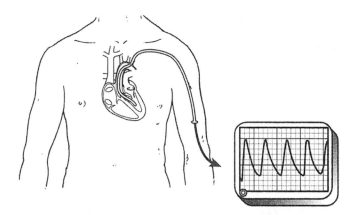

FIGURE 20–2

Catheterization of the left heart. The catheter is threaded up an artery and into the left ventricle. By comparing pressures in the left ventricle and the aorta just outside the heart, it's easy to determine if there is narrowing of the aortic valve. Special catheters can be directed into the openings of the coronary arteries so that dye can be injected into the vessels; x-ray movies can then be recorded.

Once the catheter is inside the heart, we can measure the pressure in the different chambers. It's also possible to detect stenosis of the aortic or pulmonic valves and evaluate the degree of narrowing. This is done by measuring the pressure above and below the valve. The pressure above a stenotic valve will be high and the pressure below the stenosis will be low.

By knowing the difference in pressure, the cardiologist can use a formula to calculate the actual size of the valve opening (see Fig. 9–8).

An ordinary x-ray shows only the silhouette of the heart—the outside. When dye is injected through a catheter, the insides of the chambers can be seen and precisely measured. Furthermore, if a valve is leaking, the jet of dye moving backward across the valve will give a good idea of the severity of the leak.

To estimate the pumping efficiency of the left ventricle the cardiologist can inject dye and record the volumes at the end of systole and the end of diastole. Using some simple measurements, the cardiologist then can measure the percentage of blood ejected with each beat, or the **ejection fraction.** This is the most accurate single measurement of ventricular function. Any congenital lesion can be detected and precisely quantified by catheter techniques.

Visualizing the coronary arteries is by far the most common reason for cardiac catheterization. A catheter is threaded up the aorta and into the opening of a coronary artery. Dye is injected and cineangiograms, or x-ray moving pictures, are recorded. The anatomy of the coronary arteries is displayed in precise detail.

Cardiac catheterization has been a godsend to diagnostic cardiology. Without the techniques of cardiac catheterization, modern cardiac surgery would not be possible.

Two questions emerge: Who is qualified to carry out cardiac catheterization? When should it be done?

Catheterization of the right heart is so simple that it is carried out in every major coronary care unit in the country every week. By means of flow-directed catheters, it is possible to measure pressures in the right atrium, the right ventricle, the main pulmonary artery, and the pulmonary capillaries. Any physician completing a residency in internal medicine should have acquired this skill. The vein used for access can be in the neck, the arm, or the groin.

Catheterization of the left side of the heart is more difficult and carries at least 10 times the risk of right heart catheterization. It should be carried out only by a physician who has had intensive, supervised training. Most cardiac fellowship programs now require a minimum of 6 months in the catheterization laboratory. The trainee should have performed hundreds of catheterizations under expert supervision before being judged competent.

WHO NEEDS CARDIAC CATHETERIZATION?

When corrective surgery is planned for any significant valvular or congenital heart lesion, catheterization is indicated. If the abnormality has been accurately diagnosed by other means and if surgery is not planned, there is no reason to carry out catheterization.

Second, *some* patients with coronary artery disease need catheterization. Some? Not all? Right. Some. Certainly not all. In the chapter on coronary artery disease there is some discussion about who needs coronary arteriography and who doesn't. It won't hurt to be very specific about it.

REASONS FOR CORONARY ARTERIOGRAPHY

1. *For the diagnosis of coronary artery disease when the diagnosis can't be established by any other means.* It should be understood that it's important for the patient to know whether coronary disease is present or not. (An 85-year-old patient lying quietly in bed in a nursing home doesn't really need this information. A 45-year-old executive or airline pilot does.)

2. *To define coronary disease when surgery is contemplated.* If the patient isn't a candidate for surgery, there's no point in performing the catheterization. An elderly patient with a permanently damaged heart who could not possibly withstand surgery doesn't need coronary arteriography. An older patient with stable angina pectoris controlled with medication doesn't need coronary arteriography. A 55-year-old patient who suffers from angina pectoris that comes on 2 weeks after a myocardial infarct is a prime candidate for surgery and angiography is urgently needed. As I tell interns and residents: "Unless you're prepared to undertake some corrective action such as bypass surgery or angioplasty on the basis of your findings, don't subject the patient to cardiac catheterization."

3. *To check out patients with chest pain but no other signs of coronary disease.* Every physician sees patients who present with worrisome chest pain. Again and again they're checked in the emergency room and the coronary care unit, and they always turn up negative for coronary disease. Their lives are compromised by fear of the disease and they often can't work. In these cases, coronary arteriography can clear the air once and for all and allow the patient to return to normal life. It's well worth performing even though the physician is almost certain that the results will be negative. Coronary arteriography is the only way of assuring everyone that there really is no disease and that the chest pain can be ignored.

ABUSE OF CORONARY ARTERIOGRAPHY

Many years ago I wrote a review in the *New England Journal of Medicine* entitled "The Abuse of Coronary Arteriography."[1] I checked cases all across the United States and found an appalling record of improper use of this superb diagnostic tool. Young women who could not possibly have had coronary disease, tennis players with sore shoulders that hurt only when they moved the joint, and elderly patients with mild symptoms who could not possibly have survived or benefited from cardiac surgery were among patients who had undergone cardiac catheterization.

With coronary arteriography, there's rarely any review by the other physicians on the staff; in smaller hospitals, there's often nobody qualified to do the reviewing. Medicare patients are subjected to some kind of review to make sure the procedure is appropriate, but for the private, pay-your-way patient it's no holds barred.

Remember that except for an acute myocardial infarction, there's hardly ever any emergency that requires a rush to cardiac catheterization. (Cardiogenic shock and severe, increasing crescendo angina are two other indications.)

NOTES

1. Phibbs B. The abuse of coronary arteriography. *New Engl J Med.* 1979; 301:1394–1396.

Cardiac Surgery

Forty to 50 years ago, the idea of operating on the inside of the heart was pure science fiction. Now it happens every day in every major hospital in the Western world. How this all came about is a fascinating study in the way science works: this can't happen until that's discovered, and that can't be discovered until something else is perfected, and so on. For instance, before World War II the only possible kind of heart surgery took place *outside* the heart. A patent ductus arteriosus could be closed off without invading the heart itself. The operation worked well and it wasn't dangerous.

The first attack on disease *inside* the heart was surgery for mitral stenosis. It's technically easy to insert a finger into the left atrium and break open the adhesions that hold the valve shut (Fig. 21–1). The problem was that there are practically always blood clots in the atrium when mitral stenosis is present. The first attempts at surgery were a disaster because blood clots were loosened and went floating out into the arteries like time bombs.

How to get rid of the clots? In 1941, a researcher at the veterinary school of the University of Wisconsin, Dr. Karl Paul Link, isolated a chemical that kept blood from clotting. It was called dicumarol, and it was the first substance of its kind in human history.

A Swedish physician named J. Eric Jorpes discovered another anticlotting drug, heparin. Now the way was open for heart surgery. After World War II, the operation for mitral stenosis became a standard procedure with very little risk.

Anticoagulant medication is given for a sufficient period before the operation so that there is no danger from clots. All the old clots will "organize," that is, they will be slowly disintegrated by the natural process of the body and no new ones will form.

The next technical stride was the invention of the heart–lung machine (Fig. 21–2). Perfected in the fifties and sixties, this machine takes the blood out of the superior and inferior vena cavae and bypasses the heart and lungs, returning the blood to an artery. The machine oxygenates the blood and propels it ahead into the arteries, thus performing the functions of both heart and lungs. Now the surgeon can actually cut open the heart and repair the inner structures. It's difficult to work on a beating heart, however. That problem is solved by actually stopping the heartbeat with a heavy dose of potassium or by packing the heart in slush. Either way, the heart is still and the surgeon can work precisely.

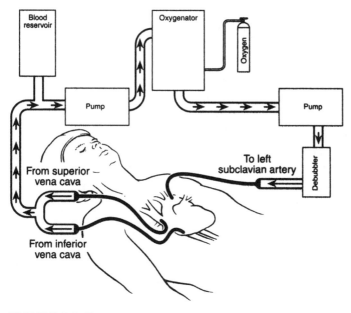

FIGURE 21-2
The heart–lung machine.

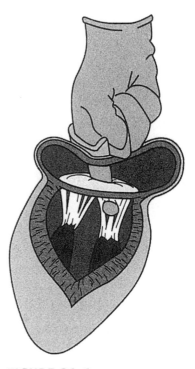

FIGURE 21-1
Closed heart operation on the mitral valve. The surgeon's index finger is inserted through an opening in the wall of the heart, and the diseased valve (mitral stenosis) is opened by gentle manipulation.

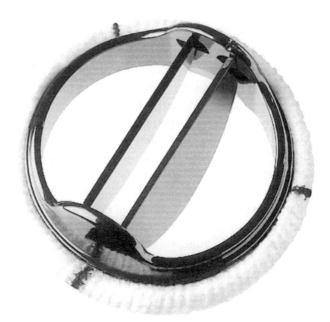

FIGURE 21-3
Prosthetic valve. The valve is made of extremely hard, long-lasting material. It consists of two flaps that open and close to mimic the action of a normal mitral valve. This "flap" type of valve is the St. Jude valve, in wide use today. (Courtesy of St. Jude Medical.)

VALVE REPLACEMENT

Artificial valves can be implanted in the mitral or aortic position. They can be made of metal and plastic or they may be actual tissue valves called **bioprostheses** that are usually from a pig (Fig. 21–3). The problem is there is always danger of clotting or infection.

The parts of a mechanical valve can wear out, and the tissue of a bioprosthesis can degenerate or calcify. The perfect valve hasn't been invented yet, but some patients have excellent results for many years—practically through a normal lifetime.

Note: There is always danger of endocarditis on an implanted valve. Endocarditis prophylaxis is particularly important. Clotting is another danger: mechanical valves should always be protected by anticoagulants. So should mitral bioprosthetic valves. The only artificial valve that doesn't present much danger of clotting is an aortic bioprosthetic valve.

Whenever a patient with an artificial heart valve suddenly shows signs of failure, assume the valve is not functioning normally. It may be stuck or it may be leaking. In either case, it's an emergency. Move fast for corrective surgery.

REPAIR OF CONGENITAL HEART DEFECTS

Septal defects can be closed with patches. Coarctation of the aorta can be repaired with a Dacron prosthesis or, in some cases, by simply cutting out the narrow area and sewing the ends of the vessel together. Practically any congenital abnormality can be corrected, partially or completely, now that the surgeon has a still, bloodless heart to work with.

CORONARY ARTERY BYPASS

It hasn't been possible to "un-harden" an artery. Once an atheromatous mass plugs up a vessel, it's there to stay. (At least until recently.)

But why not go around the obstruction? How about a detour? Dr. René Favaloro of Buenos Aires decided that might be a good idea. He took a piece of vein out of a patient's leg and grafted, or tacked, one end of it to the aorta. He then attached the other end to the coronary artery beyond the point of obstruction. The "coronary artery bypass" was thus born (Figs. 21–4 and 21–5).

Coronary artery bypass surgery is now, by far, the most common heart operation in the world. How well does it work? Who needs it? What is the risk?

If the graft system stays open, the results are good. About 20% of grafts will close within the first 6 months and about 4% more will close each year after that. That's the best anyone's been able to do. The vein grafts close because of blood clots, new atheromas, or thickening of the lining cells of the vein.

Within these limitations, coronary bypass surgery is useful in the treatment of angina. It can be counted on to relieve pain when medical measures fail; it cannot be counted on to prolong life in more than 15% of patients. Thus, coronary bypass

Pluses, Minuses, and Reasonable Expectations	
Annual mortality from coronary disease based on vessels involved:	
RCA alone	2.8%
LAD alone	4%
Circumflex alone	4%
Combination of any two of the above	7%
All three of the above	12%
LMCA alone	12%

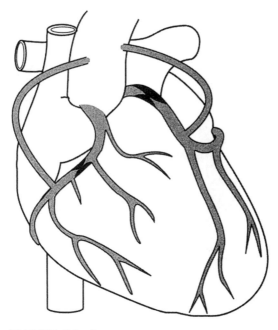

FIGURE 21–4
Principle of coronary bypass grafting. (Courtesy of
Dr. Jack Copeland, University of Arizona Medical
Center.)

surgery is a reasonable alternative when angina is so severe that it prevents a patient
from living a reasonably normal life and when medical measures have failed. Who can
expect to live longer as a result of coronary artery surgery? Obviously, the mortality
from single-vessel disease of any of the three branches is so low that it's not reasonable to expect major heart surgery to improve it, and it doesn't.

Back in Chapter 8 there's a list of conditions when, as we now know, coronary bypass
surgery can prolong life. To say it one more time, for the benefit of anyone contemplating
this procedure, cororonary artery bypass surgery can be expected to prolong life if

1. The left main coronary artery is diseased
2. The left anterior descending vessel is severely diseased near its origin and the
   function of the left ventricle is compromised
3. All three coronary arteries are severely diseased
4. Possibly in cases when two vessels are diseased and one of them is the left
   anterior descending artery with disease near its origin

In any other case, coronary bypass surgery will relieve pain. That's all.

Note: *In any other setting, coronary artery surgery offers only relief of pain. It is justified
solely if anginal pain is severe and if it cannot be controlled by medical means.*

An artery that runs along the chest can sometimes be brought down and connected to the diseased coronary artery. Grafts using the internal mammary artery are
much more satisfactory than vein grafts and are more likely to stay open. Even arterial
grafts can close off, however.

Coronary bypass surgery can succeed only if there is a localized area of hardening
with a good vessel beyond it to put the graft in. If there is diffuse hardening scattered
all along an artery it can't be bypassed.

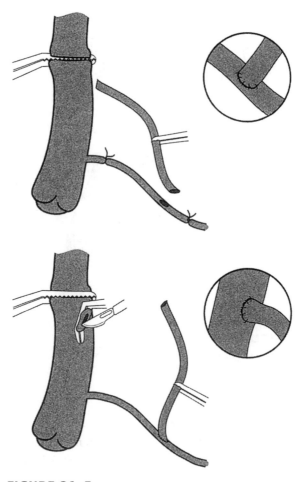

FIGURE 21–5
Technique of coronary bypass grafting. (Courtesy of
Dr. Jack Copeland, University of Arizona Medical Center.)

Unfortunately, the process of atheroma formation goes right on in the other coronary arteries. It progresses much faster in the part of the coronary arteries that has been bypassed. Most bypassed arteries are completely closed off in 6 months. Now the blood flow to that area is completely dependent on the graft. If the graft closes, the heart muscle is lost.

What's the risk of the operation? That depends on the patient. In an otherwise healthy patient with a good ventricle, the risk is about 1%. In an elderly patient with a left ventricle that isn't pumping efficiently, the risk may be as high as 10% to 15%. A second bypass operation is at least twice as risky as a first one. The risk is higher in patients who have had previous myocardial infarcts and is much higher in older patients (over 65). Simply being put on a heart–lung bypass machine for 3 or 4 hours can have serious consequences for older patients.

Note: Twenty percent of coronary bypass grafts will close off within 6 months. Disease in the bypassed vessels progresses very rapidly after bypass, and most vessels will be closed in 6 months. In other words, the risk may be so high that the operation might not be justified. Patient and cardiologist should discuss numbers like these for a long time before surgery is attempted.

CORRECTING ABNORMALITIES WITH A CATHETER

Balloon Angioplasty

It's now possible to perform operations on the inside of the heart without surgery, without the risk of cutting open the chest, and even without anesthesia. It's done with a catheter.

Andreas Gruentzig, a Swiss cardiologist, introduced a startling procedure. He made a catheter with a strong balloon at the end, threaded the catheter through a diseased coronary artery so that the balloon was exactly at the atheroma, and then inflated it. The whole idea sounds fantastic, but it works. The balloon actually "cracks" the atheroma, fracturing it and dilating the artery.

Balloon angioplasty is now part of standard operating procedure at every major medical center. After the artery has been dilated a stent, or sleeve, is threaded into the vessel to hold it open and cut down the chances of restenosis. Some of these stents have been coated with special material that, it is hoped, may further help the stent stay open. Whether these coated stents are really better than the bare metal ones is still a subject of investigation. In any case with modern stent techniques the reclosure rate is down around 15% or less.

There can still be complications, such as tearing or dissecting a vessel or actual myocardial infarction. For this reason, there has been much discussion about the safety of angioplasty in a hospital that doesn't have surgical backup. There's still divided opinion on this subject too, but my personal opinion is that except for some extreme emergency, angioplasty should be performed only where there's surgical backup immediately available and close at hand.

Does angioplasty prolong life? Is it as effective as bypass grafting? The answer to both these questions now appears to be yes—in some settings; basically the same settings as in bypass grafting.

If there is disease in many branches of the coronary arteries so that four or even five grafts are needed, bypass surgery is clearly superior to angioplasty.

There are risks and limitations, of course. Sometimes it isn't possible to reach the diseased area with a catheter. The artery may tear along its coats, or dissect, when the balloon is inflated, or the patient may actually suffer a myocardial infarction during the procedure. In either case, emergency bypass surgery must be performed.

How does angioplasty affect life expectancy in the long term? Which patients are the best candidates for angioplasty? These questions haven't been answered yet, but in properly selected cases, angioplasty certainly offers relief of anginal pain when medical management has failed. It is not known whether angioplasty prolongs life in any category of coronary disease. Studies are under way to evaluate this possibility.

Atherectomy

There are now several other methods of attack on the atheroma. One is the atherectomy approach. There have been enough complications with cutting atherectomy to ensure caution in its use. Some cardiologists still use the method while others have substantially abandoned it. The chief utility of laser treatment at this point is to open a hole in a thick atheroma so that a balloon catheter can be threaded through.

After an artery is opened by any of these means, a stent is introduced to cut down the possibility of restenosis. A specialized catheter with a cutting end can be used to dissect the atheroma and remove it. Special types of laser-tipped catheters have also been used to burn away the atheroma. The trick here is to focus the laser on the atheroma without damaging the coronary artery itself: with improvement in techniques this goal is nearer.

All these methods are being studied and improved. It's not too much to hope that some kind of direct attack on the atheroma will be successful in the not-too-distant future.

Balloon Valvuloplasty

Remember the original surgical approach to mitral stenosis? The surgeon simply put his finger in the valve and broke open the adhesions. It's possible to do the same thing with a couple of strong balloons on a catheter. The operator threads the catheter from a vein to the right atrium. A special catheter tip is then used to punch a small hole in the septum between the atria: the catheter is passed into the left atrium and down across the mitral valve. The balloons are inflated, and the scars holding the valve edges together are broken.

Balloon valvuloplasty for mitral stenosis is remarkably effective. If the valve isn't too hardened with calcium, it's certainly the best approach available today. Balloon valvuloplasty for aortic stenosis has not worked well, at least in adults, and shouldn't be tried.

Surgery of cardiac structures by means of catheters is in its infancy. The next few years are going to see an explosion of this kind of technology.

REPAIR OF AORTIC ANEURYSM

An aneurysm is a "ballooning" or progressive dilatation of the aorta that is caused by a weakening of the wall. The common cause of an aneurysm is degeneration of the wall around an atheroma (Fig. 21–6). The danger is that an aneurysm can rupture, with instantly fatal results.

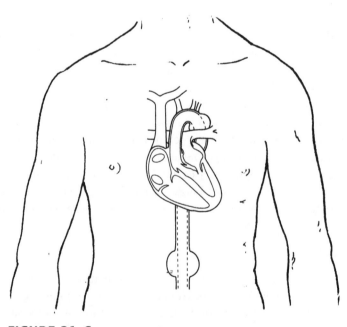

FIGURE 21–6

Aortic aneurysm. The risk of rupture depends on the size of the aneurysm. If the aneurysm is in the thoracic aorta (the part in the chest), 7 cm is the critical diameter. Any aneurysm this large should be corrected surgically. If the aneurysm is in the abdomen, the cutoff size is probably 4 cm; 6 cm in diameter certainly calls for surgery.

The only symptom produced by an aneurysm is pain. If an aneurysm becomes painful or if it increases to a critical size, prompt surgery is the only treatment. Results of surgery are excellent.

A brilliant innovation for repair of abdominal aneurysms was introduced by some cardiac surgeons at University of California, Los Angeles. Basically, a plastic tube carefully molded to fit inside the abdominal aorta is threaded up from an incision in the groin, thereby sealing off the aneurysm and providing a new, strong lining for the aorta. This technique is now used everywhere and it's been surprisingly successful.

DISSECTING ANEURYSM

The wall of the aorta can tear along its inner layer. These tears look as if someone had taken a sharp knife and made a slit in the inner coat of the aorta, without going all the way through.

Blood forces its way through this slit and tears apart the layers of the wall of the aorta, actually dissecting them apart. As the dissection progresses, a clot fills this space. Sometimes the dissection can go all the way around the arch of the aorta and on down into the part in the abdomen (Fig. 21–7).

Aortic dissection is a true medical emergency. There will always be severe pain. Often the blood pressure will be elevated. If the dissection progresses, the pain may move on down the body in a way quite different from the pain of coronary disease.

Dissection is more likely to occur in patients with inherited weakness of the connective tissues and in pregnant women. Treatment consists of prompt lowering of blood pressure to ease the strain on the wall of the aorta. Surgical correction will be

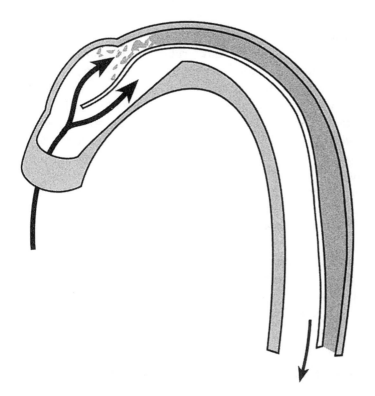

FIGURE 21–7
Dissecting aneurysm.

needed in many cases. If the dissection is limited to a defined area in the arch of the aorta or further out, medical treatment may suffice to stop the dissection and allow healing to take place.

CARDIAC TRANSPLANTATION

In 1967, Dr. Christian Barnard reported from South Africa that he had successfully transplanted a heart from a dead patient to a living one. This was one of the most startling advances in the whole history of medicine; the world was stunned. Unfortunately, the first wave of enthusiasm didn't last long. It turned out that life after transplantation was short and unpleasant. Biologists predicted a sequence of grim complications, and they were right.

The first problem was rejection. All the cells in any one body recognize each other—like members of the same tribe. When strange cells appear, they are attacked and destroyed. If cells didn't act like this, life would not be possible, since this is the basis for the body's defense against bacteria and other invaders. Without this immune system to guard the body, people would die of the first disease-causing bacteria that appeared.

The trouble is that when tissues from one person are implanted in another person's body, they are identified as foreign invaders and the immune system gears up to attack and destroy them. This is what causes rejection: the tissues of the implanted organ are literally "eaten up" by the defenses of the body they're implanted in.

There are ways of turning off this immune reaction; many drugs will do it. Trouble is, when the immune system is turned off so that the implanted organ isn't rejected, the patient has no way of fighting infection. The first transplant patients died as a result of rejection and infection and for a time in the early 1970s, the whole idea was almost abandoned.

It was back to the drawing board of basic science. Studies of the causes of rejection, better means of controlling infection and turning off the immune response, and the appearance of new agents to control viral infections all added up to a real breakthrough during the 1980s. Now cardiac transplantation can be performed with survival rates that compare favorably with many other forms of major surgery for life-threatening disease.

At the University of Arizona, Dr. Jack Copeland and his associates have been able to show a 96% survival rate at the end of 1 year and an 85% survival rate at the end of 4 years. When you consider that the transplant patients were all people who were literally dying at the time of their operations, these are remarkable numbers. Properly equipped major centers in other parts of the world have produced similar results. Artificial hearts have been invented that actually fill the role of a heart in pumping blood. The chief use of these instruments is to act as a "bridge" to maintain life while a patient waits for a heart to be transplanted. (Remember, a human heart has to be found that can be transplanted in a very short time and that heart has to match the patient's heart in some very specific ways.) These artificial hearts have been used to maintain life for surprisingly long periods—even months—until a suitable donor heart can be obtained. I'm proud to be able to report that one model has been perfected here at the University of Arizona under the leadership of our chief of cardiac surgery, Dr. Jack Copeland.

Cardiac Transplantation: The Larger Issues

Now that heart transplantation can be performed, the medical profession and society at large have some troubling questions to answer:

1. *What patients are suitable candidates for heart transplantation?* Candidates for a transplanted heart must be patients who are near death from heart disease and for whom all conventional treatments have been exhausted. The patient must have a reasonable life expectancy in terms of age and must be mentally competent to cope with the complications of life after transplantation.

2. *What patients should not receive a transplanted heart?* It would be ridiculous to implant a heart in a patient who had some other disease that couldn't be controlled or that would predictably shorten life. Emphysema, some severe forms of diabetes, many forms of infection, degenerative diseases of the liver or kidneys, and cancer are some of the conditions that make it impossible to consider cardiac transplantation. It would be equally ridiculous to implant a new heart in someone so old that life couldn't be prolonged much anyway. Most programs consider the age of 60 a cutoff point, although there are exceptions.

3. *What does the procedure cost?* There's a considerable expense. At many institutions, deposits or commitments from insurers ranging from $45,000 to over $125,000 are typical. By any standards, anywhere, cardiac transplantation is expensive.

4. *How does this expensive procedure fit into the overall financial and social structure of medical care?* At a time when the national health budget is terribly strained, the question of great expense for a relatively short-term gain becomes agonizing. Obviously, major government funding sources, like Medicare and Medicaid, can't afford many of these procedures per year. It's painful, but true: at this time, cardiac transplantation is reserved for the wealthier segments of society and there's no prospect of an immediate change.

Life after transplantation—what's it like? It's certainly much better than it used to be. Many patients go back to very strenuous activity like marathon running and gymnastics, and the great majority are physically able to resume some kind of work. Unfortunately, the enormous stress of the illness preceding transplantation and of the procedure itself seems to leave some patients mentally exhausted. One national study showed that 57.9% of transplant patients felt they could return to work, but only 25% actually did so.

Note: The techniques of transplantation have improved so dramatically in the last few years that it's reasonable to expect much better results in the near future. Cardiac transplantation today may be only a crude beginning for unimaginable vistas in the next few years.

Heart Attack

Half of all deaths are caused by disease of the heart and blood vessels. The chances are good, therefore, that you will be on hand when someone actually has a heart attack. It is a common occurrence. If the heart attack strikes on the golf course, by a fishing stream, on a ski slope, or at any place far from medical aid, what can you do? (After a lifetime of backpacking, fly-fishing, and skiing in remote areas I have a deep personal interest in this subject.)

There are only a few things that the nonmedical person can do for the victim of a heart attack. These few things, however, may be very important. There are also some things that you should *not* do.

A heart attack will be one of two things: (1) acute left heart failure or (2) some type of coronary artery syndrome.

ACUTE LEFT HEART FAILURE

The symptom of acute left heart failure will be shortness of breath. The victim will be panting very rapidly with shallow breaths, the color of his lips and earlobes may be bluish, he will refuse to lie down flat, and he will fight you if you try to force him to do so. He will be sitting up, gasping desperately for breath. He is fighting for breath because his lungs are engorged with blood, which is trapped in back of a failing left heart (Chap. 6).

What to Do

Place tourniquets as high up as you can around the patient's arms and legs. The tourniquets can be strips of cloth, heavy rubber bands, neckties, handkerchiefs, or anything that can be knotted and twisted, preferably with a stick or pencil. Tighten the tourniquets, but check to be sure you can still feel a pulse in the patient's wrists and feet.

Send for help.

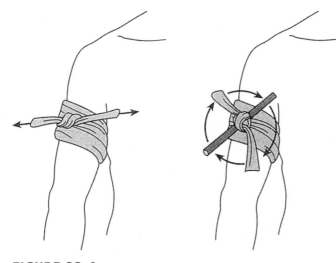

FIGURE 22–1

Treatment of left heart failure. The patient cannot breathe because the lungs are engorged with blood. Apply tourniquets as high as possible on the arms and legs. Twist the tourniquets tight until you can just feel a pulse in the wrists and feet. In 10 or 15 minutes, when the patient has begun to breathe easily, release one tourniquet. In another 15 minutes, retighten this tourniquet and loosen another. Continue rotating the tourniquets.

In about 5 or 10 minutes, the victim will begin to breathe more easily. When this happens, loosen one of the tourniquets, leaving the other three tight. Every 15 minutes, retighten the slack tourniquet and loosen another one—in other words, rotate the tourniquets (Figure 22–1).

If necessary, you can keep up this rotation of tourniquets for several hours while you wait for help to arrive. If you are really in the wilderness, days from help, you can start to release the tourniquets one at a time after a couple of hours if the patient's breathing seems easier. The tourniquets can always be reapplied, if needed.

Don't try to make the patient walk about. *Don't* throw cold water on his face. *Don't* try to give him artificial respiration. *Don't* try to make him eat or drink anything—he won't want to, and he shouldn't.

CORONARY HEART ATTACKS

These will be either angina pectoris, myocardial ischemia, or a myocardial infarct. The symptom will be pain or some other acute discomfort, usually in the front half of the upper body. The pain may be over the heart or anywhere on the front of the chest. It may go up the sides of the neck toward the jaws. It often goes down the arms, particularly the left arm. Sometimes the pain will be in the very upper part of the abdomen, just at the lower end of the breastbone. The victim may think that he has acute indigestion, and he will almost always be frightened or apprehensive.

ANGINA PECTORIS

If the patient is a known sufferer from angina pectoris, help him to take his nitroglycerin or another quick-acting coronary dilator. Help him find a place to rest, and watch him while the pain goes away. If it is a typical attack, and he is used to them, he will be able to resume activity when the pain has disappeared.

MYOCARDIAL ISCHEMIA AND MYOCARDIAL INFARCTION

The pain will not go away, even with rest or with nitroglycerin. The discomfort persists, and the patient is usually very apprehensive. You can do these things:

1. Put the patient at rest in a chair, couch, or bed. Sometimes he will want to move about and walk around in a frightened, agitated manner. Don't let him do it. Make him be quiet.
2. Relieve the pain. Aspirin, whiskey, or any of the common pain-relieving agents available are all useful. Alcohol is good because it relieves pain and calms the frightened, agitated patient.
3. Send for help. Even if this means waiting for horses, helicopters, or some other means of travel out of rugged country, don't move the patient until help arrives.

Don't move the patient about or let him move himself about; keep him quiet. *Don't* force him to eat; foods and liquids should be given in very small quantities as he desires them. *Don't* apply artificial respiration or give stimulants such as caffeine.

"STOPPAGE" OF THE HEART

Acute left heart failure or coronary disease of any kind may cause the heart to stop pumping blood. This may happen in one of two ways: the ventricles may simply stop beating and hang motionless (ventricular standstill; see Chap. 12) or the ventricles may go into a feeble twitching motion, which cannot pump any blood (ventricular fibrillation; see Chap. 12).

In either case, the patient will fall as though shot. He will be motionless and he will not breathe. He is not yet dead, and he does not really have to die in many cases. Surprisingly often his life can be saved if there is someone nearby who knows what to do.

Note: Remember, the patient is not breathing and his heart is not beating. In 3 or 4 minutes the cells of the brain will begin to die for lack of oxygen. Whatever is to be done must be done at once.

To treat stoppage of the heart, you must first decide that it has happened. **Making a diagnosis** is the first step. The diagnosis of heart stoppage rests on two simple observations:

1. The patient is not breathing.
2. He has no pulse.

It is usually easy to tell when someone is not breathing by simply looking at the chest. A hand placed on the chest will help detect very slight breathing movements.

Taking a pulse is simple, but most people do not know how to do it. Look at Figure 22–2 to see how to take the pulse in the wrist and neck. Practice on yourself and others. This is a skill that most people should possess.

Give yourself 10 seconds to make the diagnosis of stoppage of the heart. This will usually be plenty of time.

Treatment consists of two operations:

1. Artificial breathing
2. Artificial pumping of the heart

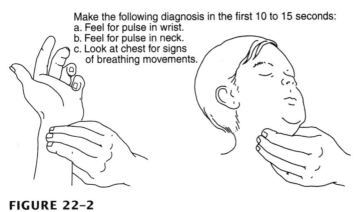

Make the following diagnosis in the first 10 to 15 seconds:
a. Feel for pulse in wrist.
b. Feel for pulse in neck.
c. Look at chest for signs
   of breathing movements.

FIGURE 22–2
Diagnose stoppage of the heart.

THE RIGHT AND WRONG WAYS TO SAVE LIVES

When the heart goes into ventricular fibrillation or stops altogether (standstill), the patient begins to die within seconds. No blood is being pumped to vital organs, principally the brain, and brain cells die very quickly when deprived of blood (within about 5 minutes, in fact).

Some years ago two brilliant physicians at Johns Hopkins University discovered that it was possible to squeeze the heart by simply compressing the chest, thus expelling enough blood to keep the patient alive. From this evolved the standard procedure of compressing the chest and breathing for the patient when the heartbeat stops. Hundreds of thousands of people have been trained in this procedure, especially those likely to be called in an emergency such as firefighters and paramedics. Standard courses are taught by the American Red Cross and the American Heart Association to train bystanders or rescuers in two maneuvers:

1. Compression of the chest to circulate blood
2. Mouth-to-mouth breathing to deliver oxygen

The previous edition of this book illustrated what was thought to be the correct way to go about this according to the standards taught everywhere. Now, thanks to the superb experimental work of two of my colleagues, Dr. Gordon A. Ewy, chief of our Cardiology Section, and Dr. Karl B. Kern, one of our senior members, the whole method of cardiopulmonary resuscitation has been changed for the better, and thousands of lives have already been saved by use of this new technique.

Here's the reasoning behind the new procedure.

First, when the heart goes into ventricular fibrillation there's a substantial reserve of oxygen in the blood—enough for 5 or possibly 10 minutes.

On the other hand, there's absolutely no blood moving through the brain and other vital organs

The first order of business is to get that blood moving, and you do it by compressing the chest. How do you compress it? Hard and fast—***100 times a minute.***

Exhaustive work on experimental animals has shown that rapid compression in that range is what's needed to generate adequate blood flow.

Figures 22–3 shows what happens to aortic and right atrial pressures during 15 chest compressions after arrest. Note that it takes a number of compressions in rapid succession to push the pressures in the vital organs up to life-sustaining levels.

Hemodynamic Response to 15 Chest
Compressions During Ventricular
Fibrillation

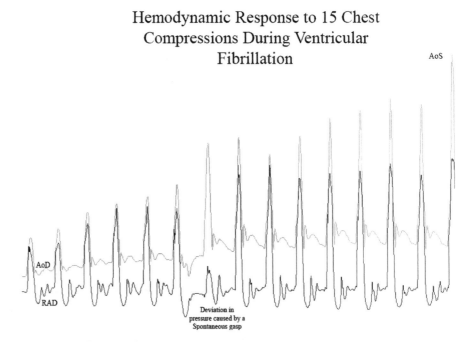

FIGURE 22–3

Simultaneous recording of aortic and right atrial pressures during
first 15 external chest compressions in swine in cardiac arrest
due to ventricular fibrillation. AoS indicates aortic "systolic"
pressure during chest compression; AoD, aortic "diastolic"
pressure during release phase; and RAD, right atrial pressure
during "diastolic" or release phase of chest compression.

Figures 22–4 through 22–6 illustrate the proper method of closed-chest massage.

That's clear enough for the first few minutes, but if the patient still isn't breathing, what then?

Sooner or later, if the patient doesn't resume breathing, someone will have to begin artificial breathing. If paramedics or firefighters arrive, breathing can be started with a simple airway and a breathing device called an *ambu* bag. If the bystander is still in charge, mouth-to-mouth breathing becomes essential. Figures 22–7 illustrates the technique of mouth-to-mouth breathing.

How often does one breathe for the patient?

That is precisely where the old standards are wrong and the new standards are lifesaving.

The old standards prescribed breathing twice between every 15 chest compressions. Careful study by the University of Arizona investigators in this country and in Wales showed that those two ventilations require at least 16 seconds by casual bystanders and 10 seconds even by skilled paramedics or other medical personnel.

Figures 22–8 illustrates what happens when chest compression is interrupted *that* often for *that* long for purposes of ventilation. There's a catastrophic fall in blood flow during the 16 seconds required for two ventilations and this fall may very well be lethal.

In other words, with the old guidelines, everybody has been ventilating too much and not compressing enough.

Extensive work with experimental animals and review of results with human subjects has shown that the new approach proposed here improves survival as much as 300%. (This new approach has been aptly termed "cardiocerebral resuscitation" since it is basically directed at supplying the brain with adequate blood.)

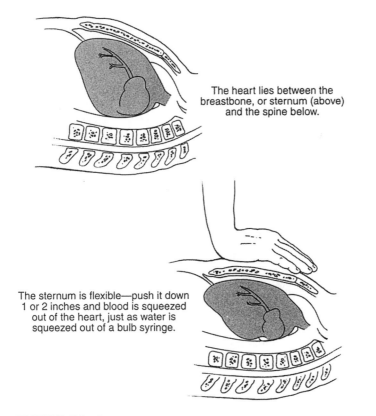

The heart lies between the breastbone, or sternum (above) and the spine below.

The sternum is flexible—push it down 1 or 2 inches and blood is squeezed out of the heart, just as water is squeezed out of a bulb syringe.

FIGURE 22–4
Perform closed-chest massage of the heart.

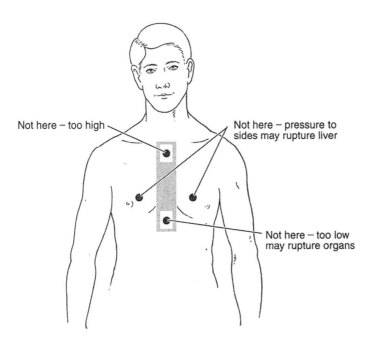

Not here – too high

Not here – pressure to sides may rupture liver

Not here – too low may rupture organs

FIGURE 22–5
Where to press to massage the heart. Press down on the main part of the sternum, shown as shaded rectangle, with the heel of the hand only. This part of the sternum starts where the ribs come together and extends up about 5 inches.

Hands are placed one over the other on the main portion of the sternum: the heel of the hand transmits the entire force.

Lean down, using the weight of your body to compress the sternum. In this way, massage can be continued almost indefinitely, whereas arm muscles used alone would soon tire.

Massage should be vigorous enough to produce a pulse in the patient's neck or wrist.

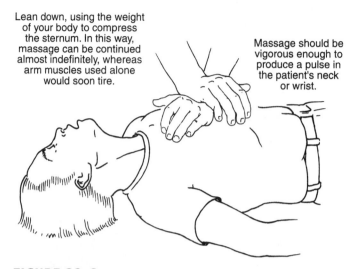

FIGURE 22–6
Closed-chest massage of the heart.

Tip head to side and empty fluid or vomit from mouth – 10 to 15 seconds.

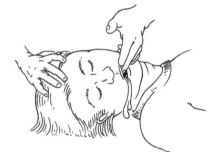

Total time so far is less than 1 minute.

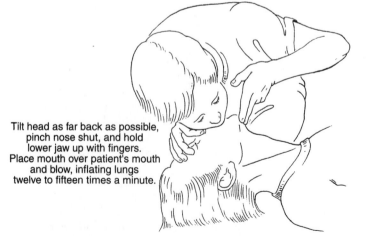

Tilt head as far back as possible, pinch nose shut, and hold lower jaw up with fingers. Place mouth over patient's mouth and blow, inflating lungs twelve to fifteen times a minute.

FIGURE 22–7
Give mouth-to-mouth resuscitation.

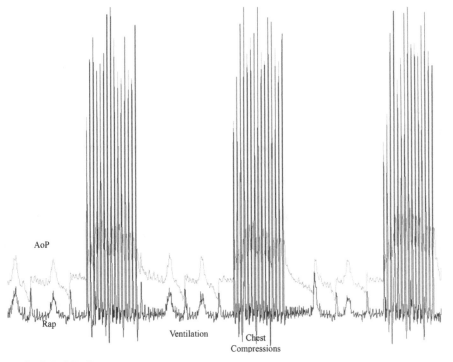

AoP

Rap

Ventilation

Chest
Compressions

FIGURE 22–8
Simultaneous recording of aortic (blue) and right atrial (yellow) pressures during
simulated single lay rescuer scenario in which each 2 ventilations are delivered within
16 seconds. ECG (bottom yellow) shows continuous ventricular fibrillation. Note that
15 chest compressions take less time than 2 ventilations.

Here are the guidelines if a victim is nonresponsive:

1. Begin chest compression promptly and vigorously at a rate of 100 per minute.

2. If a defibrillator arrives, don't let anyone halt the proceedings for defibrillation
   until at least 200 vigorous chest compressions have been completed. If the
   patient has simply been lying there without chest compression, the time required
   to attach the instrument and make a reading is likely to be lethal.

3. If there's no help and the patient isn't breathing after 4 or 5 minutes, begin
   mouth-to-mouth breathing at a rate of no more than one breath for every 100
   compressions.

4. If the bystander doesn't want to do mouth-to-mouth breathing, simple compression
   should be used until help can come. *Simple compression without ventilation has
   proved successful in several parts of the United States.*

5. Important new information: it's easy to overventilate!
   Overventilate? Is there such a thing as too much air?

Not exactly. The problem is that forced ventilation, even with a simple breathing
bag and airway, increases pressure within the chest. That increase in pressure cuts
down on the amount of venous blood returning to the heart and lungs. When those
vital organs are starved for blood anyway, this drop in circulation can be critical.

In fact, the motion of compressing the heart also compresses the lungs and produces
a certain amount of air exchange—that's one reason simple compression does so well.

With all this in mind, here are further recommendations:

When paramedics or fire department personnel arrive they should place an oropharyngeal airway—a non-rebreather mask—and begin high-flow oxygen. That's all the ventilation the patient needs, in addition to the ventilation produced as a byproduct of cardiac compression.

What's wrong with breathing with a breathing bag?

Studies by the University of Arizona investigators show that even paramedics and physicians overventilate: they seem to become so carried away with the need for oxygen that they squeeze a breathing bag too often, sometimes as often as they compress the heart! (Remember, this forced breathing is cutting down on the flow of blood back to the heart and lungs.) In other words, with standard methods, everybody's been undercompressing the heart and overventilating the lungs.

Speaking of overventilation, we now come to intubation. For the nonmedical reader, the term *intubation* means that someone opens the patient's mouth widely, depresses the tongue with a special instrument so that the vocal cords become visible, and threads a tube directly into the trachea, or windpipe. This is not easy and is sometimes impossible. Only experienced personnel with a great deal of training should even attempt this in the setting of a cardiac arrest. Delay in inexperienced hands can be and often is fatal. There's one word for endotracheal intubation in the acute stage of a cardiac arrest. DON'T. Paramedics or physicians should never attempt to intubate the patient during the acute stage of resuscitation.

First, the patient doesn't need intubation for adequate ventilation.

Second, during the effort to intubate, there's no chest compression. That means there's no blood circulating. Even a very skilled intubator will take at least 20 seconds to have a tube in the larynx and functioning. For most people it takes much longer: if the procedure requires several attempts, several minutes will be lost and so will the patient's life. (I've witnessed many attempts at intubation by unskilled physicians and heard the frantic mutter "just a minute: one more try") until I had to remove physician and intubation equipment by main force, restart compression, and ventilate with simple tube and bag.

Later, after the patient is stabilized, it may be necessary to intubate to keep up normal respiratory exchange if the patient cannot do it spontaneously. This should be done only after adequate circulation has been reestablished—in other words, after the heart is beating spontaneously to deliver an adequate volume of blood. Then the delay necessitated by intubating the trachea and beginning programmed artificial breathing won't endanger the patient's life.

Think over these steps. Have them so well memorized that you will do them no matter how many terrified amateurs are giving the wrong advice or getting in the way. Sometimes life will return in an astonishingly short time. I have seen a heart begin to beat and a patient begin to breathe within 10 seconds. It is certainly tragic to think of a human life wasted for the want of such a simple lifesaving procedure.

If the accident happens in civilized surroundings, keep going until medical aid arrives, even if this takes an hour. Many patients have lived after 2 hours of closed-chest massage and mouth-to-mouth breathing. In the wilderness, far from any possible help, you should think of an hour as the minimum time to continue the effort. In the absence of skilled medical help don't assume the patient is dead or beyond hope. However, at the end of an hour, if the patient shows obvious signs of death, it is probably time to give up.

When the patient is actually dead beyond reviving, the pupils of the eyes will become very large. The lips and nail beds and ears will all be a distinct blue color. The patient will be making no attempt to breathe on his own, and there will be no detectable pulse.

Read this section thoroughly, and, if possible, get some actual experience in closed-chest massage and mouth-to-mouth breathing in a first-aid group.

When you see such an emergency, go through the measures systematically and fast. Don't let anything stop you from going through every step just outlined.

NOTES

Ewy GA. Cardiocerebral resuscitation: the new CPR. *Circulation*. 2005;111:2134–2142.

Aufderheide TP, Sigurdsson G, Pirrallo RG, et al. Hyperventilation-induced hypotension during cardiopulmonary resuscitation. *Circulation*. 2004;109:1960.

Aufderheide TP, Lurie KG. Death by hyperventilation. *Crit Care Med.* 2004:32 (suppl):345–351.

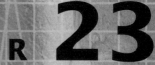

CHAPTER 23

Measuring the Efficiency of the Heart

How well is the heart performing its job of pumping blood? (**Ventricular function** is the term cardiologists use to describe the pumping efficiency of the heart.) A cardiologist must be able to answer this question before deciding whether cardiac surgery will be safe or helpful. For example, coronary artery surgery may prolong life in patients with three-vessel disease and mild depression of ventricular function. If ventricular function is normal, bypass surgery will not improve survival; if it is severely depressed, bypass surgery will be too dangerous. In a disease such as myocardiopathy, measurement of ventricular function is often the only way a cardiologist has of knowing that disease is in fact present and how serious it is.

After many false starts and a great deal of research, it is now possible to measure ventricular function very accurately.

The heart pumps about 6 liters of blood a minute. This volume is called **cardiac output.** Cardiac output is simple to measure, but it isn't a good index of ventricular function. A patient with a normal cardiac output can still die of heart failure.

Stroke volume is the amount of blood pumped out of the heart with each beat and is easy to calculate using simple arithmetic. If the heart is pumping 6,000 cc of blood per minute and beating 80 times a minute, the stroke volume will be 75 cc. This is a step further but it still doesn't give an accurate idea of cardiac function.

After many false starts, a reliable measurement of ventricular function has emerged. This measurement is called the **ejection fraction.** Everyone involved in the care of cardiac patients must know what the ejection fraction is, what the normal values are, and how these values are used (Fig. 23–1).

The ventricles pump out only part of the blood they contain with each beat. Obviously, they can't eject all the blood since that would leave a vacuum. If there are 125 cc in the left ventricle at the end of diastolic filling, about 75 cc will be ejected by a healthy ventricle—in other words, 60%. **Thus the ejection fraction is the amount of blood pumped out with each beat compared to the amount of blood that was in the**

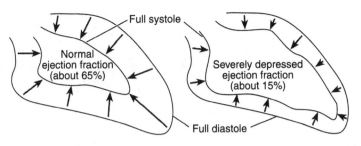

FIGURE 23–1

Measuring ejection fraction. Outline of the ventricle in systole and diastole.

ventricle to start with. To put it another way, "What percentage of the blood in the ventricle gets pumped out with each beat?"

$$Ejection\ fraction =$$
$$\frac{Volume\ at\ the\ end\ of\ diastole\ -\ Volume\ at\ the\ end\ of\ systole}{Volume\ at\ the\ end\ of\ diastole}$$

Normal ejection fraction	65% (approximately)
Depressed ejection fraction	below 50%
Seriously depressed ejection fraction	30% or below
Critically depressed ejection fraction	20% or below

The ejection fraction is the best predictor of survival in coronary artery disease. It is the most important yardstick of risk when surgery is being considered. It is, overall, the most reliable prognostic measurement in any type of heart disease.

It is a curious fact that as reliable as the ejection fraction is, it often doesn't correlate with symptoms. Thus a patient with a very depressed ejection fraction may be able to perform surprisingly well on a treadmill or in real life. Even though the heart has been severely damaged, the vascular system can often adapt amazingly well for a time.

HOW THE EJECTION FRACTION IS MEASURED

The outline of the ventricle is obtained during a whole heart cycle, so that the total size at the end of diastolic filling can be compared with size at the end of systolic emptying. This can be done during cardiac catheterization (when dye is injected into the ventricle) by two-dimensional (2-D) echocardiography, or by radioisotope methods (the MUGA scan).

The maximum and minimum ventricular sizes are then overlaid and compared; the ejection fraction can be calculated by simple measurements. Experienced cardiologists can estimate the ejection fraction with acceptable accuracy by simply looking at the two outlines.

The ejection fraction can also be measured from the 2-D echocardiogram. The cardiologist observes the beating heart in several projections and estimates the ejection fraction. There are no exact formulas: the cardiologist must assess the force of contraction in the various parts of the left ventricle and try to average them into an overall ejection fraction. While there is considerable variation between observers with this method, it works surprisingly well and in most cases correlates satisfactorily with other methods.

CHAPTER 24

Special Diagnostic Procedures

ECHOCARDIOGRAPHY

In the book and movie *The Hunt for Red October*, each side found the other's submarines underwater by bouncing sound waves off them. The same principle is used in modern medical diagnosis: sound waves of a certain frequency are projected through part of the body. When the sound waves are reflected off certain organs or tissues, these reflections (or echoes) form a pattern that can be recognized. It's possible to see a fetus in the uterus, outline gallstones, and detect abnormalities in the shape and size of many organs.

Echocardiography uses this technique to outline the structures of the heart. In addition, the echoes give a continuing picture so that the moving, beating heart can be seen and its motion analyzed.

There are two methods of displaying the echocardiogram. The older method, called M-mode display, gives a view through one narrow segment of the heart—the "icepick" view (Fig. 24–1).

Later the two-dimensional (or 2-D) method was developed. With the aid of computers, an image of the heart can be projected as if it were a motion picture (Fig. 24–2).

Speed of blood flow within the heart can be calculated by the Doppler phenomenon: reflected sound waves from red blood cells moving toward and away from a particular spot are recorded and the speed of blood flow through that area can be measured. Blood will move abnormally fast through a narrowed area—such as a stenotic aortic valve—and by measuring the speed above and below the valve, it's possible to calculate the exact degree of narrowing. Abnormal motion of blood, such as the backward flow when valves leak, can also be detected. The Doppler probe is shown in Figure 24–3.

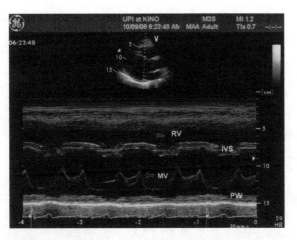

FIGURE 24-1

M-mode echocardiogram. This was the earliest form of echo recording. A narrow beam is directed down through the heart and successive beats are recorded. From the top down: the anterior wall of the right ventricle (RV), the right ventricular cavity, the interventricular septum (IVS), the anterior and posterior leaflets of the mitral valve, and the posterior ventricular wall (PW). (Courtesy of Migvel Acosta, Chief Technologist, heart lab, University/Kino Hospital.)

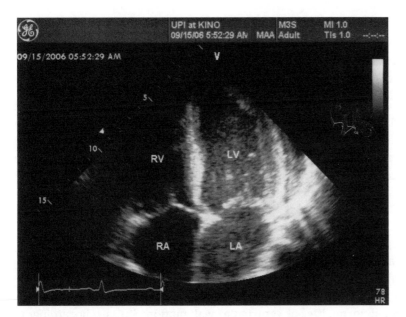

FIGURE 24-2

2-D or two-dimensional echocardiogram. The heart is shown upside down and backward. RV = right ventricle, LV = left ventricle, RA = right atrium, LA = left atrium. The left-sided chambers are clearly defined with a cloudy mass of echo-generating material (Optison) that has been injected in a vein and is now moving through the heart. (Courtesy of Migvel Acosta, Chief Technologist, heart lab, University/Kino Hospital.)

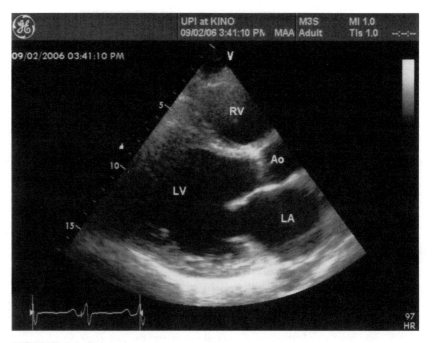

FIGURE 24-3

Echocardiogram recorded from the left sagittal view. This means that the patient lying flat and the echocardiogram is recorded so that you are looking at the heart "sideways," that is, from the left side of the chest. RV = right ventricle, LV = left ventricle, Ao = aorta, LA = left atrium. (Courtesy of Migvel Acosta, Chief Technologist, heart lab, University/Kino Hospital.)

What Is Echocardiography Used for and When Should It Be Used?

- **Measurement of chamber size:** Echocardiography should give exact measurements. This is especially important for the evaluation of valvular disease such as aortic insufficiency or mitral stenosis.
- **Observation of wall motion and measurement of ejection fraction:** The 2-D echo makes it possible to see dead, scarred areas of the ventricle that don't move normally. Calculation of ejection fraction by 2-D echo is usually accurate enough for all clinical purposes.
- **Visualization of the structure and motion of the heart valves:** This can be critical to the evaluation of valvular stenosis or regurgitation (Fig. 24–4).
- **Diagnosis of congenital lesions:** Echocardiography has been particularly valuable in this field. In many cases, it's so precise that it isn't necessary to catheterize the heart to establish the diagnosis.
- **Detect abnormalities of ventricular wall motion:** Stress echocardiograms recorded during and after exercise may be able to pick up abnormalities of motion of the ventricular wall that indicate an inadequate blood flow. This is still experimental, but it's promising.

Echocardiograms are not able to record the anatomy of the coronary arteries, and they can't help in the diagnosis of myocardial infarction. Experiments are under

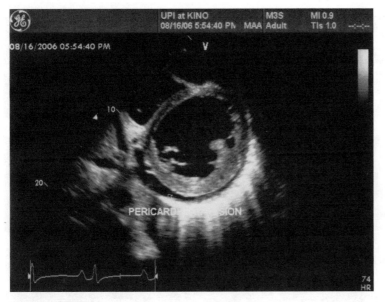

FIGURE 24–4

This is the short-axis or "cross-cut" viewing the heart. This is taken as if a cut had been made across the middle of the heart allowing the physician to look directly at the tissues as if they really had been sliced to permit viewing. The almost-round ring of tissue is the wall of the left ventricle. The dark space around it, as indicated, is pericardial fluid. (Courtesy of Migvel Acosta, Chief Technologist, heart lab, University/Kino Hospital.)

way at some major medical centers to see if it's possible to detect very small changes in wall motion that might indicate an infarct, but so far the results are indefinite.

RADIOISOTOPE METHODS

The use of radioactive thallium has been described in Chapter 8 on coronary artery disease. It makes stress testing more accurate in some selected cases. A very useful application of radioisotope methods is the MUGA or multiple gated acquisition. A radioisotope is injected that tags the red blood cells. As the blood moves through the heart, the radioactivity is measured by very sensitive detectors. These detectors are triggered by the electrocardiogram so that recordings are synchronized with the heart cycle. It is possible to outline the chambers of the heart very accurately and to see the movement of the heart through the whole heart cycle (Fig. 24–5).

Measurement of the ejection fraction is very precise with good MUGA equipment. It's also possible to see abnormalities of wall motion and to detect valvular regurgitation, but these are less important functions. Knowing the ejection fraction, the cardiologist can decide if coronary bypass surgery is justified or if it will be safe. When myocarditis or myocardiopathy is suspected, a depressed ejection fraction together with abnormal wall motion gives critical information about diagnosis and prognosis. All this can be accomplished with a completely safe, painless test. It's not surprising

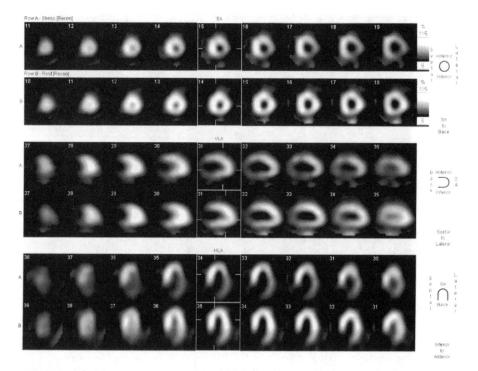

FIGURE 24–5

Stress and rest myocardial perfusion images in a 63-year-old male with pain in chest and left neck upon exertion. Images were obtained after sepmate injections of Tc-99m tetrofusmin at peak exercise and at rest. Matched stress and rest tomographic images of the left ventricle are shown (top to bottom) in short-axis, vertical long-axis, and horizontal long-axis projections. Stress images show decreased radiotracer activity in the lateral and inferolateral left ventricular wall; these regions are normal on rest images, consistent with stress-induced myocardial ischemia. Stress electro-cardiogram was nondiagnostic for stress-induced ischemia. The patient underwent coronary artery bypass surgery 2 weeks later with subsequent resolution of symptoms.

that cardiologists regard the MUGA technique as one of the great advances of the last few decades.

Newer techniques include nuclear magnetic resonance and gated CT scans that are triggered by the electrocardiogram. There are still ferocious arguments about technique, but it seems likely that both methods will be useful in the future.

Review Test

1. The chambers that make up the heart are called the _____ and the _____.

2. The right heart consists of the _____ and the _____. The left heart consists of the _____ and the _____.

3. Blood returning from the veins of the body flows into the _____, then to the _____, the _____, the _____, the _____, and the _____, and finally out through the _____.

4. The two great veins that empty all the blood of the body into the right atrium are called the _____ and the _____.

5. The blood moves from the right heart into the lungs through the _____.

6. The blood moves from the lungs to the left atrium through the _____.

7. The blood moves out of the left ventricle to the body through the _____.

8. There is an inlet valve and an outlet valve for each ventricle. The valve that swings open to let the blood flow from the right atrium into the right ventricle is called the _____. The valve that swings open to let the blood flow from the left atrium to the left ventricle is called the _____.

9. The outlet valve from the right ventricle is called the _____. The outlet valve from the left ventricle is called the _____.

10. The layers of the heart from the outside in are the _____, the _____, and the _____.

11. When a heart chamber contracts, squeezing the blood forward, it is called _____. When it relaxes and fills again, it is called _____.

12. The blood supply of the heart structures comes through the _____. There are four main branches of these vessels, called the _____, the _____, the _____, and the _____.

13. When the ventricles contract, raising the pressure of the blood inside them, the _____ and _____ valves open. At the same time, the _____ and

_____ valves close. When the ventricles relax to fill with blood in diastole, the _____ and _____ valves open, and the _____ and _____ valves close.

14. Like all muscle, the heart muscle can contract only when it is stimulated by an electric impulse through nerve or nervelike tissue. The electric impulse that makes the heart beat is formed in the _____. This electric impulse then moves down through the _____ and across the _____. The waves produced when the electric impulse moves across the atria are called _____. The waves produced during activation of the ventricles are called _____, _____, and _____ waves.

15. The function of the heart is to deliver _____ to the tissues of the body.

16. When blood moves through the lungs, it picks up oxygen from the air cells, or _____. Blood coming back from the body to the lungs carries a waste product called _____. This is breathed out at the same time the oxygen is breathed in. Blood can carry oxygen because of a chemical called _____ in the red blood cells.

17. When congestive heart failure occurs, fluid may pile up in two locations in the lungs: in the _____ or, more dangerously, in the _____. There is only one symptom of congestive heart failure—_____.

18. The term *edema* means _____.

19. A dangerous form of congestive heart failure that occurs when masses of fluid pile up in the alveoli is called _____.

20. Right heart failure means that the blood cannot get out of the right heart and into the lungs as fast as the veins return it to the right atrium. Right heart failure produces only one symptom, namely, _____ of the _____, or lower, parts of the body.

21. The major organs where catastrophe strikes as a result of hypertension are the _____, the _____, and the _____.

22. Certain natural chemicals circulate in the body with the function of causing the smaller arteries to constrict in order to adjust the fluid state of the body to various challenges. These chemicals are called _____; they are formed at the _____ and in the _____.

23. There are four general categories of antihypertensive drugs; these are the _____, the _____, the _____ and the _____.

24. Accelerated or malignant hypertension is characterized by _____, _____, and _____ or _____, and, in 50% of cases, by _____.

25. Abrupt rise in blood pressure with symptoms of cerebral or cardiac involvement is called hypertensive crisis. Which of the following statements is true?

Hypertensive crisis is best treated by reassurance and some adjustment of medicine. _____

Hypertensive crisis should prompt the physician to search for psychic trauma and other sources of mental stress. _____

26. The one drug safe and appropriate to use in a hypertensive crisis is _____.

27. Abrupt appearance of hypertension in an older patient raises the possibility of _____, a specifically curable entity.

28. Two rare but curable types of hypertension are associated with diseases of the
_____.

29. Coronary artery disease may present in one of four typical clinical patterns:
_____, _____, _____, or _____.

30. What percent of patients with myocardial infarction die before reaching a hospital?
_____%.

31. The causes of death associated with myocardial infarction are _____
_____, or _____.

32. The electrocardiogram will always be abnormal early in the course of myocardial
infarction. If the electrocardiogram is normal, the patient can safely be discharged.

True ___ False ___

33. The diagnosis of myocardial infarction is established by two kinds of objective
tests: _____ and _____.

34. Crescendo angina is almost always caused by a clot forming in the diseased
portion of a coronary artery; anticoagulant treatment with heparin should always
be part of management.

True ___ False ___

35. Coronary arteriography should be carried out whenever coronary artery disease
is suspected.

True ___ False ___

36. Coronary bypass surgery can be expected to improve the pumping action of the
ventricle.

True ___ False ___

37. **Multiple choice:** Coronary arteriography should

   a. always be carried out immediately after thrombolytic therapy of myocardial
   infarction.

   b. routinely be carried out a week or so after thrombolytic therapy of infarction.

   c. be carried out only in selected cases after thrombolytic therapy—namely, in
   those patients with persistent pain after 24 hours, recurrent angina, or poor
   exercise treadmill performance after the infarct has healed.

   Answer(s): _____

38. The symptoms associated with aortic stenosis are _____, _____,
_____, or _____.

39. The 2-year mortality following appearance of these symptoms is _____%.

40. The danger of aortic regurgitation is that it can produce severe enlargement and
failure of the left ventricle. If this has gone on too long, even replacement of the
valve does not halt the downward course.

True ___ False ___

41. Mitral stenosis and mitral insufficiency both produce one symptom, namely
_____.

42. Tricuspid regurgitation is almost always the result of left heart failure with elevation
of pulmonary artery and RV pressures.

True ___ False ___

43. In the Western world, myocarditis is usually caused by a(n) _____.

44. The diagnosis of myocarditis is usually based on exclusion of other causes of impaired cardiac function.

True ___ False ___

45. Before the discovery of penicillin, the mortality of bacterial endocarditis was _____%.

46. Endocarditis can form around any structural abnormality in the heart, including _____ or _____.

47. Endocarditis is preventable. A patient with any abnormality that can lead to endocarditis should receive antibiotic prophylaxis before any surgery or instrumentation of any body cavity—oral, genital, or anal.

True ___ False ___

48. Multiple choice: Mitral valve prolapse is

    a. a very serious disease that always requires diagnostic study catheterization and intensive medical management.

    b. a harmless anomaly in over 99% of cases. There's no risk to the patient and no major diagnostic studies or cardiac medications are needed or justified. In more severe cases, endocarditis prophylaxis may be indicated.

    Answer(s): _____

49. In the adult heart, the minimum time required for an impulse to leave the sinus node, traverse the atria and the AV node–His bundle complex, and reach the ventricles is _____ second. The same passage should never take longer than _____ second.

50. The time required for the activating impulse to traverse the ventricular network is normally _____ second or less.

51. A pathologic Q wave is defined as one that is _____ second in width.

52. The "quiet part" of the heart cycle, when the current of injury produced by damaged heart muscle will show up, is called the _____ segment.

53. The electrocardiogram records enlargement of the chambers of the heart with a high degree of accuracy.

True ___ False ___

54. The ST deviation of pericarditis differs from the deviation of myocardial infarction in one important respect: _____.

55. At best, exercise stress testing will be about ___% accurate; there are both false-positive and false-negative errors.

56. Two sources of error that can invalidate stress testing are _____ with _____ and _____.

57. If a patient can't walk enough to perform an exercise stress test, two variations of the method are _____ and _____.

58. Sinus arrhythmia is a harmless change in rhythm that comes and goes with _____.

59. Ectopic beats may arise in the _____, the _____, or the _____.

60. If a ventricular complex is narrow (0.10 second or less), it must arise in the _____ of the heart—that is, in the _____ or in the _____.

61. If an ectopic beat arises in the ventricles, it will never be less than _____ second wide.

62. Define the word *paroxysmal*.

_____.

Now define the word *tachycardia*.

_____.

What do the two terms mean when combined?

_____.

63. If a paroxysmal tachycardia produces narrow ventricular complexes, it must arise in the _____ or the _____.

64. Ventricular tachycardia will always produce ventricular complexes that are at least _____ second wide.

65. Ventricular tachycardia is almost always associated with significant heart disease and is often dangerous.

True ___ False ___

66. When the ventricles are responding to fibrillating atria, the ventricular rhythm will always, without exception, be irregular.

True ___ False___

67. The immediate danger of atrial fibrillation is _____. A long-term danger is

_____.

68. The complications of atrial flutter are the same as the complications of atrial fibrillation—namely, congestive heart failure—because of the rapid rate or the discharge of blood clots.

True ___ False ___

69. The common symptoms of the sick sinus syndrome are _____, caused by inadequate blood flow to the brain, and _____.

70. The bradycardia-tachycardia syndrome is a combination of two disorders of rhythm. They are _____ and _____.

71. True sick sinus syndrome is rare; "false" sick sinus syndrome produced by drugs or vagal effect is common.

True ___ False ___

72. First-degree heart block means that there's a consistent, one-to-one PR relation: the PR interval is over _____.

73. In the Wenckebach type of AV nodal block, the PR intervals before the blocked beat get progressively _____. The PR interval in the first beat after the blocked beat always _____.

74. Type I (Wenckebach) block is practically always found in the _____. Type II block (Mobitz type II) is practically always found in the _____.

75. In type II block, the PR intervals before and after the blocked P wave are

_____.

76. There are three criteria for the diagnosis of complete heart block. They are _____, _____, and _____.

77. The two fatal arrhythmias are _____ and _____.

78. A form of ventricular fibrillation often caused by drugs is called _____. It is associated with _____.

79. The most common form of congenital heart disease is _____.

80. An atrial septal defect is relatively benign; a ventricular septal defect, if large, is much more serious.

   True ___ False ___

81. The Eisenmenger syndrome is most commonly caused by a(n)_____ or a(n)_____.

82. Severe hypertension in a young individual should always raise suspicion of _____.

83. Aortic stenosis may lead to sudden cardiac death. So can one other congenital heart lesion, namely, _____.

84. Some congenital lesions that produce cyanosis at birth require urgent surgical correction. One example is _____.

85. Be sure you understand the difference between the pink puffer and blue bloater types of COPD. What are the blood oxygen levels in each? _____

86. The normal stimulus to breathing is the _____.

87. The stimulus to breathing in the severe COPD blue-bloater patient is the _____.

88. Breathing high levels of oxygen can be dangerous in COPD because _____.

89. Right heart failure in COPD is caused by _____.

90. The simplest, safest, and quickest treatment of pulmonary edema is _____.

91. The second step in treating pulmonary edema is always _____.

92. Steps 3 and 4 are _____ and _____.

93. Is digitalis a powerful or relatively weak agent in treatment of acute heart failure? _____.

94. Is the blood volume in congestive heart failure always increased or decreased? _____.

95. Drugs that lower preload include _____ and _____.

96. Drugs that lower afterload include _____, _____, and _____.

97. Oxygen is of little help in treatment of severe chronic congestive heart failure.

   True ___ False ___

98. _____% of coronary bypass grafts must be expected to close within the first 6 months after surgery. _____% must be expected to close every year after that.

99. Coronary artery bypass surgery can be expected to prolong life in all categories of coronary disease.

   True ___ False ___

100. Coronary artery bypass surgery may prolong life in the following groups of patients:

   a. _____

   b. _____

   c. _____

101. The risk of a first coronary bypass procedure is about 1% in an otherwise healthy patient. Factors that increase the risk are _____, _____, and _____.

102. Balloon valvuloplasty is remarkably effective for _____. It is not effective or safe for _____.

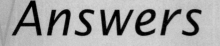

Answers

1. The chambers that make up the heart are called the <u>atria</u> and the <u>ventricles</u>.

2. The right heart consists of the <u>right atrium</u> and the <u>right ventricle</u>. The left heart consists of the <u>left atrium</u> and the <u>left ventricle</u>.

3. Blood returning from the veins of the body flows into the <u>right atrium</u>, then to the <u>right ventricle</u>, the <u>pulmonary artery</u>, the <u>lungs</u>, the <u>left atrium</u>, and the <u>left ventricle</u>, and finally out through the <u>aorta</u>.

4. The two great veins that empty all the blood of the body into the right atrium are called the <u>superior vena cava</u> and the <u>inferior vena cava</u>.

5. The blood moves from the right heart into the lungs through the <u>pulmonary artery</u>.

6. The blood moves from the lungs to the left atrium through the <u>pulmonary veins</u>.

7. The blood moves out of the left ventricle to the body through the <u>aorta</u>.

8. There is an inlet valve and an outlet valve for each ventricle. The valve that swings open to let the blood flow from the right atrium into the right ventricle is called the <u>tricuspid valve</u>. The valve that swings open to let the blood flow from the left atrium to the left ventricle is called the <u>mitral valve</u>.

9. The outlet valve from the right ventricle is called the <u>pulmonic valve</u>. The outlet valve from the left ventricle is called the <u>aortic valve</u>.

10. The layers of the heart from the outside in are the <u>epicardium</u>, the <u>myocardium</u>, and the <u>endocardium</u>.

11. When a heart chamber contracts, squeezing the blood forward, it is called <u>systole</u>. When it relaxes and fills again, it is called <u>diastole</u>.

12. The blood supply of the heart structures comes through the <u>coronary arteries</u>. There are four main branches of these vessels, called the <u>left main artery</u>, the <u>left anterior descending</u>, the <u>circumflex</u>, and the <u>right coronary artery</u>.

13. When the ventricles contract, raising the pressure of the blood inside them, the <u>aortic</u> and <u>pulmonic</u> valves open. At the same time, the <u>mitral</u> and <u>tricuspid</u> valves

close. When the ventricles relax to fill with blood in diastole, the <u>tricuspid</u> and <u>mitral</u> valves open, and the <u>pulmonic</u> and <u>aortic</u> valves close.

14. Like all muscle, the heart muscle can contract only when it is stimulated by an electric impulse through nerve or nervelike tissue. The electric impulse that makes the heart beat is formed in the <u>sinoatrial node</u>. This electric impulse then moves down through the <u>atrioventricular node</u> and across the <u>bundle branch system</u>. The waves produced when the electric impulse moves across the atria are called <u>P waves</u>. The waves produced during activation of the ventricles are called <u>Q</u>, <u>R</u>, and <u>S</u> waves.

15. The function of the heart is to deliver <u>oxygen</u> to the tissues of the body.

16. When blood moves through the lungs it picks up oxygen from the air cells, or <u>alveoli</u>. Blood coming back from the body to the lungs carries a waste product called <u>carbon dioxide</u>. This is breathed out at the same time the oxygen is breathed in. Blood can carry oxygen because of a chemical called <u>hemoglobin</u> in the red blood cells.

17. When congestive heart failure occurs, fluid may pile up in two locations in the lungs: in the <u>interstitial tissues</u> or, more dangerously, in the <u>alveoli</u>. There is only one symptom of congestive heart failure—<u>shortness of breath</u>.

18. The term *edema* means <u>watery swelling of tissues</u>.

19. A dangerous form of congestive heart failure that occurs when masses of fluid pile up in the alveoli is called <u>pulmonary edema</u>.

20. Right heart failure means that the blood cannot get out of the right heart and into the lungs as fast as the veins return it to the right atrium. Right heart failure produces only one finding, or sign, namely, <u>edema</u> of the <u>dependent</u>, or lower, parts of the body.

21. The major organs where catastrophe strikes as a result of hypertension are the <u>brain</u>, the <u>heart</u>, and the <u>kidneys</u>.

22. Certain natural chemicals circulate in the body with the function of causing the smaller arteries to constrict in order to adjust the fluid state of the body to various challenges. These chemicals are called <u>catecholamines</u>; they are formed at the <u>sympathetic nerve endings</u> and in the <u>adrenal glands</u>.

23. There are four general categories of antihypertensive drugs; these are the <u>catecholamine-blocking drugs</u>, the <u>ACE inhibitors</u>, the <u>beta blockers</u>, and the <u>calcium blockers</u>.

24. Accelerated or malignant hypertension is characterized by <u>elevated diastolic pressure</u>, <u>retinal charges</u>, and <u>cerebral</u> or <u>cardiac symptoms</u>, and, in 50% of cases, by <u>kidney failure</u>.

25. Abrupt rise in blood pressure with symptoms of cerebral or cardiac involvement is called hypertensive crisis. Which of the following statements is true?

Hypertensive crisis is best treated by reassurance and some adjustment of medicine. <u>False</u>

Hypertensive crisis should prompt the physician to search for psychic trauma and other sources of mental stress. <u>False</u>

26. The one drug safe and appropriate to use in a hypertensive crisis is <u>nitroprusside</u>.

27. Abrupt appearance of hypertension in an older patient raises the possibility of <u>renal artery stenosis</u>, a specifically curable entity.

28. Two rare but curable types of hypertension are associated with diseases of the <u>adrenal glands</u>.

29. Coronary artery disease may present in one of four typical clinical patterns: <u>typical (Heberden's) angina pectoris</u>, <u>Prinzmetal angina</u>, <u>crescendo angina</u>, or <u>myocardial infarction</u>.

30. What percent of patients with myocardial infarction die before reaching a hospital? <u>50</u>%.

31. The causes of death associated with myocardial infarction are <u>cardiac arrest</u>, <u>cardiogenic shock</u>, or <u>congestive heart failure</u>.

32. The electrocardiogram will always be abnormal early in the course of myocardial infarction. If the electrocardiogram is normal, the patient can safely be discharged. True ___ False __✓__

33. The diagnosis of myocardial infarction is established by two kinds of objective tests: <u>electrocardiogram</u> and <u>measurement of cardiac enzymes in the blood</u>.

34. Crescendo angina is almost always caused by a clot forming in the diseased portion of a coronary artery; anticoagulant treatment with heparin should always be part of management. True __✓__ False ___

35. Coronary arteriography should be carried out whenever coronary artery disease is suspected. True ___ False __✓__

36. Coronary bypass surgery can be expected to improve the pumping action of the ventricle. True ___ False __✓__

37. **Multiple choice:** Coronary arteriography should

    a. always be carried out immediately after thrombolytic therapy of myocardial infarction.

    b. routinely be carried out a week or so after thrombolytic therapy of infarction.

    c. be carried out only in selected cases after thrombolytic therapy—namely, in those patients with persistent pain after 24 hours, recurrent angina, or poor exercise treadmill performance after the infarct has healed.

    Answer(s): <u>b and c are both considered as possibilities.</u>

38. The symptoms associated with aortic stenosis are <u>dizziness</u>, <u>fainting</u>, <u>shortness of breath</u>, or <u>angina</u>.

39. The 2-year mortality following appearance of these symptoms is <u>50</u>%.

40. The danger of aortic regurgitation is that it can produce severe enlargement and failure of the left ventricle. If this has gone on too long, even replacement of the valve does not halt the downward course. True __✓__ False ___

41. Mitral stenosis and mitral insufficiency both produce one symptom, namely, <u>shortness of breath</u>.

42. Tricuspid regurgitation is almost always the result of left heart failure with elevation of pulmonary artery and RV pressures. True __✓__ False ___

43. In the Western world, myocarditis is usually caused by a <u>virus</u>.

44. The diagnosis of myocarditis is usually based on exclusion of other causes of impaired cardiac function. True __✓__ False ___

45. Before the discovery of penicillin, the mortality of bacterial endocarditis was <u>100</u>%.

46. Endocarditis can form around any structural abnormality in the heart, including <u>diseased valves</u> or <u>congenital defects</u>.

47. Endocarditis is preventable. A patient with any abnormality that can lead to endocarditis should receive antibiotic prophylaxis before any surgery or instrumentation of any body cavity—oral, genital, or anal. True __✓__ False ___

48. **Multiple choice:** Mitral valve prolapse is

   a. a very serious disease that always requires diagnostic study catheterization and intensive medical management.

   b. a harmless anomaly in over 99% of cases. There's no risk to the patient and no major diagnostic studies or cardiac medications are needed or justified. In more severe cases, endocarditis prophylaxis may be indicated.

   Answer: b

49. In the adult heart, the minimum time required for an impulse to leave the sinus node, traverse the atria and the AV node–His bundle complex and reach the ventricles is 0.12 second. The same passage should never take longer than 0.20 second.

50. The time required for the activating impulse to traverse the ventricular network is normally 0.10 second or less.

51. A pathologic Q wave is defined as one that is 0.04 second in width.

52. The "quiet part" of the heart cycle, when the current of injury produced by damaged heart muscle will show up, is called the ST segment.

53. The electrocardiogram records enlargement of the chambers of the heart with a high degree of accuracy. True _ False __✓__

54. The ST deviation of pericarditis differs from the deviation of myocardial infarction in one important respect: there is never ST depression with pericarditis.

55. At best, exercise stress testing will be about 75% accurate; there are both false-positive and false-negative errors.

56. Two sources of error that can invalidate stress testing are medication with digitalis and preexcitation.

57. If a patient can't walk enough to perform an exercise stress test, two variations of the method are dobutamine echo and Persantine thallium.

58. Sinus arrhythmia is a harmless change in rhythm that comes and goes with breathing.

59. Ectopic beats may arise in the atria, the AV node, or the ventricles.

60. If a ventricular complex is narrow (0.10 second or less), it must arise in the top half of the heart—that is, in the atria or in the AV node.

61. If an ectopic beat arises in the ventricles, it will never be less than 0.12 second wide.

62. Define the word *paroxysmal*.

   Anything that stops and starts abruptly.

   Now define the word *tachycardia*.

   Any rate over 100.

   What do the two terms mean when combined?

   Paroxysmal tachycardia means a rapid regular beat that starts and stops abruptly.

63. If a paroxysmal tachycardia produces narrow ventricular complexes, it must arise in the atria or the AV node.

64. Ventricular tachycardia will always produce ventricular complexes that are at least 0.12 second wide.

65. Ventricular tachycardia is almost always associated with significant heart disease and is often dangerous. True __✓__ False ___

66. When the ventricles are responding to fibrillating atria, the ventricular rhythm will always, without exception, be irregular. True __✓__False ___

67. The immediate danger of atrial fibrillation is <u>congestive heart failure</u>. A long-term danger is <u>blood clots with embolization</u>.

68. The complications of atrial flutter are the same as the complications of atrial fibrillation—namely, congestive heart failure—because of the rapid rate or the discharge of blood clots. True __✓__ False ___

69. The common symptoms of the sick sinus syndrome are <u>vertigo</u> and <u>syncope</u>, both caused by inadequate blood flow to the brain.

70. The bradycardia-tachycardia syndrome is a combination of two disorders of rhythm. They are <u>periods of supraventricular tachyarrhythmia (fibrillation, flutter, or tachycardia)</u> and <u>periods of significant slowing of the sinus node</u>.

71. True sick sinus syndrome is rare; "false" sick sinus syndrome produced by drugs or vagal effect is common. True __✓__ False ___

72. First-degree heart block means that there's a consistent, one-to-one PR relation: the PR interval is over <u>0.20 second</u>.

73. In the Wenckebach type of AV nodal block, the PR intervals before the blocked beat get progressively longer. The PR interval in the first beat after the blocked beat always <u>shortens</u>.

74. Type I (Wenckebach) block is practically always found in the <u>AV node</u>. Type II block (Mobitz type II) is practically always found in the <u>bundle branches</u>.

75. In type II block, the PR intervals before and after the blocked P wave are <u>the same</u>.

76. There are three criteria for the diagnosis of complete heart block. They are <u>complete AV dissociation, a slow ventricular rate (45 or less)</u>, and <u>no capture or conducted beats despite an adequate number of atrial complexes to test the system</u>.

77. The two fatal arrhythmias are <u>ventricular fibrillation</u> and <u>ventricular standstill</u>.

78. A form of ventricular fibrillation often caused by drugs is called <u>torsades de pointes</u>. It is associated with <u>rapidly changing QRS morphology with 180° changes in axis</u>.

79. The most common form of congenital heart disease is <u>bicuspid aortic valve</u>.

80. An atrial septal defect is relatively benign; a ventricular septal defect, if large, is much more serious. True __✓__ False ___

81. The Eisenmenger syndrome is most commonly caused by a <u>ventricular septal defect</u> or a <u>patent ductus arteriosus</u>.

82. Severe hypertension in a young individual should always raise suspicion of <u>coarctation of the aorta</u>.

83. Aortic stenosis may lead to sudden cardiac death. So can one other congenital heart lesion, namely, <u>pulmonic stenosis</u>.

84. Some congenital lesions that produce cyanosis at birth require urgent surgical correction. One example is <u>complete transposition of the great vessels</u>.

85. Be sure you understand the difference between the pink puffer and blue bloater types of COPD. What are the blood oxygen levels in each? <u>Blood oxygen levels are normal in the pink-puffer patient and depressed in the blue-bloater patient</u>.

86. The normal stimulus to breathing is the <u>carbon dioxide level in the blood</u>.

87. The stimulus to breathing in the severe COPD blue-bloater patient is the <u>oxygen level in the blood</u>.

88. Breathing high levels of oxygen can be dangerous in COPD because <u>the stimulus to breathing is removed and the patient can go into a coma caused by inadequate breathing activity</u>.

89. Right heart failure in COPD is caused by <u>an abnormally high resistance to the flow of blood from the right heart into the lungs</u>.

90. The simplest, safest, and quickest treatment of pulmonary edema is <u>rotation of tourniquets</u>.

91. The second step in treating pulmonary edema is always <u>intravenous furosemide</u>.

92. Steps 3 and 4 are <u>oxygen</u> and <u>morphine</u>.

93. Is digitalis a powerful or relatively weak agent in treatment of acute heart failure? <u>Digitalis is a relatively weak agent in treatment of acute heart failure</u>.

94. Is the blood volume in congestive heart failure always increased or decreased? <u>The blood volume in congestive heart failure is always increased</u>.

95. Drugs that lower preload include <u>nitroglycerin</u> and <u>furosemide</u>.

96. Drugs that lower afterload include <u>nitroprusside</u>, <u>hydralazine</u>, and <u>ACE inhibitors</u>.

97. Oxygen is of little help in treatment of severe chronic congestive heart failure.
    True ___ False __✓__

98. <u>20</u>% of coronary bypass grafts must be expected to close within the first 6 months after surgery. <u>4</u>% must be expected to close every year after that.

99. Coronary artery bypass surgery can be expected to prolong life in all categories of coronary disease.
    True ___ False __✓__

100. Coronary artery bypass surgery may prolong life in the following groups of patients:
    a. <u>patients with left main disease</u>
    b. <u>patients with three-vessel disease and moderate depression of left ventricular function</u>
    c. <u>some patients with two-vessel disease that includes the left anterior descending artery</u>

101. The risk of a first coronary bypass procedure is about 1% in an otherwise healthy patient. Factors that increase the risk are <u>depression of left ventricular function</u>, <u>age</u>, and <u>complicating disease such as diabetes</u>.

102. Balloon valvuloplasty is remarkably effective for <u>mitral stenosis</u>. It is not effective or safe for <u>aortic stenosis</u>.

Notes for Coronary Intensive Units

This appendix covers some specific points of clarification and emphasis in the field of critical care.

RIGHT AND LEFT HEART PRESSURES: THE SWAN-GANZ CATHETER

To understand what you're measuring with a Swan-Ganz catheter, you have to understand one term—left ventricular end-diastolic pressure, or LVEDP. Picture the heart at the end of diastole. The mitral valve is still wide open. The flow of blood into the ventricle has stopped. The ventricle is completely filled. Everything is in a momentary pause before the next systole.

This pause is called the end-diastolic period. By measuring the pressure in the ventricle at this point, you can tell whether the heart is failing or not.

The left heart is said to fail when it can't pump the blood out into the arteries as fast as blood runs in from the lungs. In other words, there's too much blood rushing in for the pumping capacity of the heart; the heart can't keep up. This usually happens because the pumping action of the heart is weakened by any of the diseases described in the book.

Whenever the pumping action of the heart is weakened, the ejection fraction will fall. Instead of pumping out about 60% of the blood it holds at the end of filling, it may pump out 40%, or 30%, or 20%—or even less. As a result, there will be too much blood left in the ventricle at the end of systole because the weakened heart muscle can't get it out.

With the next heart cycle, a normal volume of blood comes rushing in from the lungs during diastole. When this is added to the abnormally large amount of blood left over from the previous systole, the pressure in the ventricle has to rise. There's nowhere else for the blood to go; an abnormally large volume of blood is locked in the ventricle and the pressure has to go up.

The time this pressure is measured, of course, is at the end of filling—at the end of diastole. Therefore, an abnormally high LVEDP means a failing left ventricle.

A normal LVEDP means that the ventricle isn't failing. A normal LVEDP means that the volumes of blood entering and leaving the heart are the same. The heart is keeping up with the inrush of blood by pumping the same amount out into the arteries.

If the LVEDP is low, the volume of fluid returning to the heart is inadequate. This can happen for a variety of reasons—dehydration, hemorrhage, septic shock, and so on.

Thus, the patient with a high LVEDP needs less fluid, and the one with a low LVEDP needs more.

How can you measure LVEDP? You can't put a catheter in the left ventricle, after all—at least not in the coronary care unit. As you know, it's easy to thread a catheter into any major vein and float it through the right heart and into the pulmonary artery. From this position, it's possible to measure the LVEDP. Here's why:

When the catheter is wedged firmly into a pulmonary capillary, it only registers the pressure ahead of it. In other words, there's a clear channel down the pulmonary veins and through the left atrium into the left ventricle. At the end of diastolic filling, pressures are equalized all the way back from the left ventricle through the left atria and on up the pulmonary veins and into the pulmonary capillaries. There are no valves in between and so, at the end of diastolic filling, the pulmonary capillary pressure, or "wedge" pressure, will be the same as the LVEDP.

Diastolic pressure in the pulmonary artery will almost always equal the wedge pressure. Always check by inflating the Swan-Ganz balloon to see if these two pressures are the same when the catheter is first inserted. If they are, you can use the pulmonary artery diastolic pressure as the wedge and you can avoid repeated balloon inflations, which can be hazardous. Have a competent cardiologist show you the differences in configuration between RA, RV, PA, and wedge waveforms. Always beware of the "false wedge," in which the tracing shows a slowly rising straight line when the balloon is inflated. This means that the tip of the catheter has been pressed against the side of the pulmonary artery, and a false pressure is being recorded.

Swan-Ganz catheters should usually not be left in place more than 3 days. Infection is always a hazard when foreign bodies are left in place for long periods.

In the past few years there has been some seriously misleading nonsense written about the Swan-Ganz catheter implying that use of this catheter increased the risk of death. When one asks the authors of these articles precisely how a catheter in this position would be dangerous, there's only a blank stare in reply and some mumbling about statistics. In fact, properly used, the Swan-Ganz catheter does not pose a risk of any kind. Two rules apply:

1. Never leave a Swan-Ganz catheter in position more than 3 days (instructions from Dr. Swan himself).
2. When first introducing the catheter, check the wedge pressure with a balloon if necessary and then see if the pulmonary artery diastolic pressure is the same as the wedge. If it is, use pulmonary artery diastolic pressure as your guide to LVEDP and don't inflate the balloon anymore. Too much inflation of the balloon can in fact lead to rupture of a pulmonary arteriole with catastrophic results.

OLDER ANTIARRHYTHMIC DRUGS

Quinidine

Therapeutic blood levels range from 4 to 8 or from 2 to 5 micrograms per milliliter (µg/mL) according to the laboratory technique used. There is very poor correlation between blood levels and therapeutic effect or toxicity. Always observe for clinical or ECG evidence of toxicity, regardless of blood levels.

Note: Quinidine should be used with caution in cases involving

- *congestive heart failure*
- *older patients*
- *renal failure*
- *AV block*
- anticoagulant therapy

Signs of Toxicity

1. Prolonged QT intervals. It should be noted that simple prolongation of the QT interval is not evidence of toxicity. There is almost always some QT prolongation when quinidine is administered.
2. Widened P waves.
3. PR prolongation.
4. QRS widening. (QRS widening should not exceed 25% of control value, that is, width of QRS before therapy started.)
5. Hypotension.

Digitalis

Therapeutic levels are 1 to 3 μg/mL for digoxin and 10 to 30 μg/mL for digitoxin.

Note: Digitalis should be used with caution in cases involving

- *older patients*
- *renal failure*
- *hypoxia*
- *patients with low potassium levels (Be alert for patients taking potassium-wasting diuretics!)*

Signs of Toxicity

1. Gastrointestinal disturbances (anorexia, nausea, vomiting)
2. Visual disturbances
3. Cardiac effects
   a. Acceleration of ectopic firing with premature beats, accelerated junctional or ventricular rhythms, or paroxysmal tachycardia. (This accelerated ectopic firing may arise from the atria, the junction, or the ventricles.)
   b. Depression of sinus node function, sometimes with sick sinus performance.
   c. Depression of AV conduction with any type of AV block.
4. *Any* paroxysmal tachycardia in a digitalized patient should be regarded as digitalis-toxic until proven otherwise.

The combination of paroxysmal atrial tachycardia with AV nodal block is almost always the result of digitalis toxicity in the setting of low-serum potassium.

Procainamide

Therapeutic levels range from 3.4 to 10 mg/mL.

Note: Same as for quinidine.

Signs of Toxicity

The signs are very similar to those of quinidine toxicity. There is a greater incidence of premature beats, paroxysmal tachycardia, flutter, and fibrillation.

Chief Hazard

Hypotension associated with intravenous administration is the chief hazard. Always monitor the blood pressure closely and always have a pressor agent ready to administer by drip.

Lidocaine

Therapeutic levels range from 3.4 to 10 μg/mL.

Note: Lidocaine should be used with caution in cases involving

- *liver disease*
- *renal failure*
- *congestive heart failure*
- *AV block (particularly complete AV block or block with Stokes-Adams episodes)*
- *SA block*
- *IV block*
- *sensitivity to procaine derivatives*

Signs of Toxicity

Conduction delay anywhere, of any type (SA, intraventricular) indicates toxicity.

CNS Symptoms

Convulsion is the primary symptom, but occasionally there may be hearing loss and paresthesia.

A comment about lidocaine. When lidocaine is given soon after an infarct, it's important to reach a stable blood level quickly and to maintain it. The best way to do this is to follow the protocol developed by Dr. Koch-Weser. Give a 100-mg bolus and start a 2-mg/min drip. After 18 minutes, give a second 100-mg bolus. Continue the drip.

The advantage of this method is that it raises the blood level of lidocaine to a therapeutic level in a few seconds. Lidocaine disappears so quickly that the level would fall below the effective range within 20 to 30 minutes—long before the continuous drip would have a chance to raise the blood level to the safety zone. The second bolus covers the gap; by the time this dose is gone, the blood level should be stable.

Calcium Blockers

These can be useful in slowing atrioventricular conduction during atrial fibrillation or flutter. But, remember that they are also excellent antihypertensive agents. They can and do drop blood pressure!

Dihydropyridine calcium blockers like amlodipine are very useful in control of hypertension and in some arrhythmias. However, verapamil, the first calcium blocker to be employed, has one frightening drawback: it is one of the most powerful negative inotropes known. In simple language, it depresses the myocardium, sometimes dangerously. In the early days of verapamil use I have seen patients go into frank pulmonary edema from the effect of verapamil. There are times when the physician might want to depress myocardial contractility—such as hypertrophic cardiomyopathy—but otherwise I can't think of any reason to use verapamil instead of safer calcium blockers.

NEWER ANTIARRHYTHMIC DRUGS

Newer antiarrhythmic drugs include mexiletine, sotalol, disopyramide, flecainide, amiodarone, and ibutilide.

Mexiletine and flecainide are used for ventricular arrhythmias but they are in fact more toxic and less effective than procainamide or quinidine. Propafenone is about equivalent to these last two drugs in effectiveness and toxicity.

Sotalol is also used for ventricular arrhythmias and has been the subject of study for conversion of atrial arrhythmias. The rate of successful cardioversion of atrial fibrillation is much lower than that with quinidine or procainamide and the risk of dangerous side effects is much higher. It has also been used to maintain sinus rhythm after cardioversion in which role it is moderately effective. In treatment or prevention of ventricular arrhythmias the drug is about as effective as quinidine or procainamide with about the same level of toxic side effects.

Amiodarone is the new antiarrhythmic drug that is a real contribution. Given IV for ventricular fibrillation it is often lifesaving. The same is true of the dangerous type of ventricular tachycardia—that is, the type that drops blood pressure and may threaten life. A dose of 120 mg is given IV with a fairly slow "push" and then followed by maintenance doses. (Remember! It takes a week of 800 mg per day to reach a sustained level. Anything less than that is useless.) Amiodarone is not very effective for conversion of atrial fibrillation to sinus rhythm but it is probably the best and safest drug available for maintainance of sinus rhythm once cardioversion has been effected.

The chief toxic effect of ibutilide is torsade—that is, potential sudden death. It may be the most dangerous drug in this regard.

Phenytoin

Therapeutic levels range from 10 to 18 mg/mL. There is really only one solid indication for the use of phenytoin in treatment of arrhythmias: ventricular ectopic activity caused by digitalis toxicity. Digitalis-toxic ventricular tachycardia is the indication par excellence for phenytoin. It is best given by the Bigger protocol—100 mg per 5 minutes, "push," until one of three endpoints is reached: that is, termination of the arrhythmia, a total dose of 1 g, or signs of toxicity. Phenytoin will also eliminate random VPCs when they are caused by digitalis toxicity.

Note: Phenytoin should be used with caution in cases involving

- *serious liver disease*
- *anticoagulant therapy*
- *low blood pressure*
- *congestive heart failure*
- *severe AV block*

Severe liver disease or anticoagulant therapy may interfere with the metabolism of phenytoin so that ordinary therapeutic doses may produce toxic levels in the blood.

Signs of Toxicity

1. AV or IV block
2. Fatal arrhythmia (ventricular standstill)
3. Bradycardia

CNS Symptoms

Chiefly, there are cerebellar symptoms, including ataxia, nystagmus, diplopia, slurring of speech, tremors, and vertigo.

NITROGLYCERIN: LIFESAVING OR LIFE-THREATENING?

A patient comes to an emergency room with pain suggestive of a myocardial infarct. A physician administers 1/150 g of nitroglycerin sublingually. The pulse falls to 30, the pressure to 60/0, and the patient almost dies. This is what my interns call "bottoming out" from nitroglycerin. Samuel Levine described the phenomenon in the 1940s and concluded that sublingual nitroglycerin should never be given in the setting of myocardial infarction.

"Wait a minute!" come the objections. "I've given lots of sublingual nitroglycerin for the pain of infarction and most of the time nothing of the sort happened. Sometimes it relieved the pain."

Correct. What nitroglycerin does depends on the hemodynamic state of the patient at the moment. Its effects can vary dramatically. Sometimes nitroglycerin can dilate coronary arteries. If the artery is chalky-hard and calcified, of course, nothing is going to dilate it; the diseased artery won't dilate, the healthy ones will, and the blood will be diverted to other areas—the phenomenon of "steal."

One thing nitroglycerin always does is to dilate the veins of the body with an acute drop in the quantity of blood entering the left ventricle. This drop in blood volume lowers the pressure in the left ventricle at the end of filling—the LVEDP.

Remember the Frank-Starling curve? The heart muscle is like a rubber band—the more you stretch it, the harder it snaps. The higher the LVEDP, the more the heart muscle is stretched and the harder it contracts.

This increasing strength of cardiac contraction with rising LVEDP is described by the Frank-Starling curve. It can't rise forever, of course. When the LVEDP reaches about 18 mm Hg, that's as much stretch as the muscle can handle. Above that point, increasing the pressure doesn't increase the force of the heartbeat. Rises in LVEDP above 18 mm Hg are totally harmful because they force more fluid from the blood into the lungs and they don't increase the force of the heart beat.

Now compare two patients with myocardial infarcts. One is a 65-year-old with hypertensive heart disease in chronic congestive heart failure. The LVEDP is usually high, and at the time of the infarct it rises to 24 mm Hg—the range of pulmonary edema. You administer nitroglycerin and the LVEDP falls. The congestive failure improves and the heart muscle can get along with less blood because the pressure on the wall of the ventricle is lower. The coronary vessels may dilate. The nitroglycerin is totally helpful.

The next patient is a 45-year-old male in excellent physical condition with an LVEDP of 12 mm Hg. The nitroglycerin drops the LVEDP to 6 or 8 mm Hg and the cardiac output falls by as much as 50%—the patient is sliding down the Frank-Starling curve. This drop in output turns on some abnormal vagal reflexes; the pulse and blood pressure fall to critically low levels. Any benefit of the nitroglycerin in dilating the coronaries is far outweighed by the hemodynamic catastrophe.

Right Ventricular Infarction and Nitroglycerin

There's one class of myocardial infarct where nitroglycerine is really disastrous and that's an infarct that involves the right ventricle. We now know that if very much of the muscle of the right ventricle is infarcted, the ability of that ventricle to pump an adequate volume of blood into the lungs is compromised. To keep the blood pressure up in this group of patients it's necessary to pump in large quantities of fluid—just the opposite of what one would do if the right ventricle were not involved. The volume of fluid presented to the heart is called "preload" so in medical jargon when the right ventricle is infarcted we say that the patient is "preload dependent." In plain English, that means that when the right ventricle is weakened, it takes a lot more fluid (blood) to get an adequate supply from the right ventricle into the lungs. For that reason, all guidelines state the following: **Nitroglycerin should never be given to an infarct involving the right ventricle. The reason is that nitroglycerin actually lowers the amount of blood returning to the right ventricle and therefore lowers the amount reaching the lungs.**

Which infarcts are likely to involve the right ventricles?

Inferior ones: Infarcts that show infarct changes in leads II, III, and avf.

If a patient presents with an inferior infarct and low blood pressure the proper procedure is to try a fluid challenge of about 50 cc of intravenous fluid and see how the blood pressure responds. If it rises with the fluid challenge it means that the right ventricle is infarcted and the patient needs large quantities of fluid.

(None of this was really understood in the days of the great Samuel Levine. He just noticed that nitroglycerine made some infarct patients a lot worse, and how right he was!)

Other rules about nitroglycerin in myocardial infarction:

1. If the patient is in failure—that is, if the LVEDP is elevated—nitroglycerin can be given in any form safely.

2. If the patient is not in failure, abrupt lowering of a normal LVEDP can be catastrophic. Never give sublingual nitroglycerin to these patients. IV nitroglycerin is safer because it is more gradual, and even then there can be hypotensive responses.

3. If a patient becomes bradycardic and hypotensive from the effects of nitroglycerin, give atropine; the abnormal reflexes are mediated through the vagus.

4. Sometimes physicians prescribe intravenous nitroglycerin to lower arterial blood pressure. It's not a good choice. The effect of the drug on arterial pressure is weak and inconstant. For acute, controlled lowering of blood pressure use nitroprusside.

CURRENT NOTES ON ANTICOAGULANTS

Heparin and Coumadin have been around for a long time, but new information about when they should be used and for what continues to emerge. Here are some relevant notes.

Should heparin be used after thrombolytic therapy for myocardial infarction? The answer depends on which therapy you're using. Heparin should always be administered immediately after t-PA: to fail to do so is to lose much of the thrombolytic effect. On the other hand, there is no evidence to show that heparin is of any benefit after streptokinase. Many physicians administer it on the basis of a therapeutic hunch, but all available controlled data suggest that there is no benefit from heparin in this setting.

Should heparin be given for myocardial infarction without thrombolysis? If the infarct is large and anterior and if it produces significant wall-motion abnormality, heparin may help reduce the risk of embolization from a mural thrombus at the site of the infarct. In any other type of infarction, there is no demonstrable benefit from the isolated administration of heparin.

Heparin should always be administered for crescendo angina. It is now clear that true crescendo angina is always a result of a clot forming in a diseased artery; heparin is an essential part of treatment. How long should it be continued? There are no definite guidelines, but three or four days would seem to be a logical minimum period.

When atrial fibrillation has been chronic—that is, present for more than about 2 weeks—Coumadin should always be administered before cardioversion. Effective anticoagulant therapy should be maintained for three weeks before cardioversion, if possible. Risk of postconversion embolization is high if the patient goes back into atrial fibrillation. Anticoagulation should be maintained for 4 months after cardioversion.

Atrial flutter presents as least as high a thromboembolic risk as atrial fibrillation. This well-documented fact tends to be overlooked by inexperienced cardiologists, but any sustained atrial flutter is an indication for Coumadin therapy. Some recent publications have tended to minimize the risk of embolization from atrial flutter, but the older cardiac literature and the experience of a whole generation of cardiologists leaves no doubt that the embolic risk of sustained flutter is substantial. All of us who treated severe rheumatic valvular disease 40 or 50 years ago are all too familiar with this hazard, and a recent study by a New Zealand cardiologist has reconfirmed it. The current confusion probably arises from the fact that flutter is often transient and is easily cardioverted—hence, many cardiologists have never in fact seen sustained atrial flutter.

Aspirin is a potent antiplatelet drug. It should always be discontinued ten days before any major surgery. If it isn't, bleeding complications can be catastrophic.

AUSCULTATION

The stethoscope can give life-or-death information in the coronary care unit. Any competent coronary care nurse should know how to listen to a heart and interpret the findings. Three specific sets of skills are essential:

1. Detection and characterization of gallops
2. Detection and characterization of murmurs, especially those of acute onset
3. Detection of rubs

First, buy a good stethoscope! The lightweight models in common use are almost useless for cardiac auscultation. A study at the University of Colorado revealed that one popular lightweight model is infact a little less sensitive than Laennec's first wooden monaural model, designed in the late eighteenth century! A good stethoscope should have heavy tubing with narrow orifices, a well-machined, heavy headpiece, and tightly fitting earpieces. Excellent models have been designed by Proctor Harvey and by Aubrey Leatham.

Gallops

Atrial Gallop or Fourth Heart Sound

This is a low-frequency sound caused by atrial systole. It comes just ahead of the first heart sound. To time it, put your finger on the carotid and note the upstroke of the pulse. A fourth heart sound will come just ahead of the carotid upstroke since it is a presystolic sound.

Filling Gallop or Third Heart Sound

This sound takes place at the end of the stage of rapid ventricular filling, as the mass of blood settles into the ventricle. It will come after the second heart sound. Again, when there's any question about which is the first heart sound, use the arterial pulse to identify it.

Significance

Many normal adults will have a fourth heart sound. If one appears suddenly or is very loud, it is significant. Either there is too much fluid volume in the ventricle, as in heart failure, or the ventricle has lost its "give" or "compliance." In either case, atrial systole makes a booming sound, as if one tapped a taut drum.

A third heart sound in the adult is always a bad sign. On the other hand, it is normal in children and adolescents An S_3 gallop in an adult indicates massive overload of the left ventricle for some reason. This may mean that there's actually too much blood, as in valvular regurgitation, or it may mean that pumping function is critically reduced by heart muscle damage.

The abrupt appearance of a third heart sound is always a grave sign, and skilled cardiologic assessment should be invoked urgently. This is especially true in the setting of a myocardial infarct or crescendo angina.

Murmurs

Systolic murmurs can be classed into one of two types—ejection or regurgitant. The vast majority of murmurs are of the ejection type, like the murmur of aortic stenosis. They start shortly after the first heart sound and stop before the second heart sound.

Regurgitant murmurs start with the first heart sound and go all the way through systole to the second heart sound. They are also called pansystolic or holosystolic murmurs.

There is no way to learn to distinguish between these two types of murmurs except to practice. Have a competent cardiologist demonstrate both at every opportunity.

The differential diagnosis of a holosystolic murmur is simple:

1. Mitral regurgitation
2. Tricuspid regurgitation
3. Ventricular septal defect

Note: When a pansystolic murmur appears in the course of a myocardial infarction it means a catastrophe. Either the mitral valve is leaking because the papillary muscle is torn or a hole has ruptured through the interventricular septum. Immediate skilled care is needed, and cardiac surgery will probably be necessary. The mortality in either case is very high.

Since the coronary care nurse will be the one in position to detect this murmur, the moral is obvious—learn to listen to murmurs and classify them!

Rubs

A pericardial rub is the sound caused by a roughened pericardium moving to and fro. In the typical form it has three components, one systolic and two diastolic, like a gruff-voiced dancing master saying ONE-two-three, ONE-two-three. When there is some bloody exudate on the epicardium, a rub will often appear on the second or third day of an infarct. As the pericarditis subsides, the rub may diminish to two sounds and sometimes even to one. Again, there's no substitute for experience in learning to characterize these sounds.

SUMMARY

These are a few notes organized in response to past questions posed by experienced coronary care personnel in the Tucson region. One should further point out that coronary care health-team members, to perform adequately, must know a great deal about specialized aspects of cardiac care, electrocardiographic diagnosis, use of antiarrhythmic drugs, and details of management involved in administering such potentially lifesaving agents as dopamine and nitroprusside. In brief, they must know more about certain aspects of acute cardiac care than the average physician who is not a trained cardiologist. This rather awesome responsibility implies that cardiac care personnel are committed to a lifetime of advanced study, attending seminars, reviewing current literature, and frequent consultations with attending physicians. Whenever this responsibility seems overwhelming, however, the cardiac care health team can reflect that they are the key to the intelligent use of coronary care techniques that have resulted in one of the first great reductions in mortality in what the late Dr. George Griffith aptly termed "the black death of the twentieth century."

Abbreviations and Acronyms Commonly Used in Cardiovascular Nursing

ABE	Acute bacterial endocarditis
ACE inhibitors	Angiotensin-converting enzyme inhibitors
ADH	Antidiuretic hormone
ADLs	Activities of daily living
AMI	Acute myocardial infarction
ASD	Atrial septal defect
AV	Atrioventricular
BP	Blood pressure
bpm	Beats per minute
CABG	Coronary artery bypass graft
CAD	Coronary artery disease
CBC	Complete blood count
CCU	Coronary care unit
CHF	Congestive heart failure
CI	Cardiac index
CO	Cardiac output
CPK	Creatinine phosphokinase
CPR	Cardiopulmonary resuscitation
C-T ratio	Cardiothoracic ratio
CVP	Central venous pressure
DOE	Dyspnea on exertion

DVT	Deep vein thrombosis
ECG	Electrocardiogram
EST	Exercise stress test
HCM	Hypertrophic cardiomyopathy
Hct	Hematocrit
HDL	High-density lipid
Hgb	Hemoglobin
HR	Heart rate
HTN	Hypertension
IABP	Intra-aortic balloon pump
ICS	Intercostal space
IE	Infective endocarditis
JVD	Jugular venous distention
JVP	Jugular venous pulse
LA	Left atrium; left atrial
LAD	Left anterior descending
LBBB	Left bundle branch block
LDH	Lactate dehydrogenase
LDL	Low-density lipid
LOC	Level of consciousness (loss of consciousness)
LSB	Level sternal border
LV	Left ventricle; left ventricular
LVEDP	Left ventricular end-diastolic pressure
LVH	Left ventricular hypertrophy
MAP	Mean arterial pressure
MCL	Modified chest lead
MI	Myocardial infarction
MRI	Magnetic resonance imaging
MVo$_2$	Myocardial oxygen consumption
MVP	Mitral valve prolapse
NTG	Nitroglycerin
PA	Pulmonary artery
PAC	Premature atrial contraction
PAP	Pulmonary artery pressure
PCWP	Pulmonary capillary wedge pressure
PND	Paroxysmal nocturnal dyspnea
PT	Prothrombin time
PTCA	Percutaneous transluminal coronary angioplasty
PTT	Partial thromboplastin time
PVC	Premature ventricular contraction
PVR	Pulmonary vascular resistance
RA	Right atrium; right atrial
RAP	Right atrial pressure
RBBB	Right bundle branch block

RCA	Right coronary artery
RV	Right ventricle; right ventricular
RVH	Right ventricular hypertrophy
SA	Sinoatrial
SBE	Subacute bacterial endocarditis
SOB	Shortness of breath
SVR	Systemic vascular resistance
VAD	Ventricular assist device
VHD	Valvular heart disease
VLDL	Very-low-density lipid
VSD	Ventricular septal defect
WBC	White blood cell

NORMAL QT INTERVALS

TABLE C-1	Normal QT Intervals by Rate and Sex		
Heart Rate	**Lower Limit**	**Upper Limit**	
		Men and Children	**Women**
40	0.42	0.49	0.50
43	0.39	0.48	0.49
46	0.38	0.47	0.48
48	0.37	0.46	0.47
50	0.36	0.45	0.46
52	0.35	0.45	0.46
55	0.34	0.44	0.45
57	0.34	0.43	0.44
60	0.33	0.42	0.43
63	0.32	0.41	0.42
67	0.31	0.40	0.41
71	0.31	0.38	0.41
75	0.30	0.38	0.39
80	0.29	0.37	0.38
86	0.28	0.36	0.37
93	0.28	0.35	0.36
100	0.27	0.34	0.35
109	0.26	0.33	0.33
120	0.25	0.31	0.32
133	0.24	0.29	0.30
150	0.23	0.28	0.28
170	0.22	0.26	0.26

Based on the studies of Lepeshkin as later expanded by Ashman and Hull.

Index

Numbers followed by the letter f *indicate figures; numbers followed by the letter* t *indicate tables.*

Abbreviations and acronyms, 216–218
Aberrant conduction, 114–116, 114f, 115f
Accelerated or malignant hypertension, 35–36
ACE (angiotensin-converting enzyme) inhibitors, 33
  effects, 36t
  side effects, 37t, 40, 161
  to treat heart failure, 161
  to treat myocardial infarction, 60
Acute left heart failure, 157–160
  first aid for, 178–179
  rotating tourniquets treatment, 157–158, 157f, 178–179, 179f
  seriousness of, 159–160
  symptom of, 178
  treatment of, 157–160
Acute pulmonary edema, 23
Adenosine, 96
Adrenal glands, 32, 32f
Adrenal hypertension, 39
Adrenaline, 31, 77
Adrenocortical adenoma, 39
Afterload
  defined, 160
  lowering, 161
Aldomet, side effects of, 37t
Aldosterone, 35
Alpha-methyldopa (Aldomet), 37t
Alpha-receptor blockers, 33, 36t

Alveoli, 18–19, 18f, 19f
Amiodarone
  side effects of, 97, 99
  to treat atrial fibrillation, 99, 211
  to treat paroxysmal tachycardia, 96
  ventricular standstill and, 112
Amlodipine, 210
Anemia, 20
Aneurysm
  dissecting, 175–176, 175f
  repair of, 174–175, 174f
Angina (chest "pain"), 37, 40, 179, *See also* Crescendo angina; Prinzmetal angina
Angina pectoris, 41–46, 44f
  characteristics of, 45t
  diagnosis of, 50, 50f, 51f
  medical management of, 56–57, 58f
  "stable," 62
  symptoms of, 43, 45–46
Angiogram, 54f, 62
Angioplasty, 61–62
Angiotensin I, 30
Angiotensin II, 30, 34f
Angiotensin-receptor blockers (ARBs), 161
Antibodies, 132
Anticoagulants, 213–214
  research on, 168
  risk factors in pregnancy, 140
  to treat atrial fibrillation, 99, 100

Aorta
    aneurysm repair, 174–175, 174f
    blood flow through, 5f
    coarctation of, 127, 127f
    dissection of, 175–176, 175f
Aortic regurgitation, 68, 68f
Aortic stenosis, 65–67, 66f
    congenital, 120–121
    symptoms of, 120, 121
Aortic valve, 6
    bicuspid, 120, 121f
Arrhythmias, 90–119
    aberrant conduction, 114–116, 114f, 115f
    atrial fibrillation, 97–100
    atrial flutter, 100–102, 101f
    atrioventricular block, 103–106, 104–106f
    complete heart block, 107–109, 108f
    drug treatment of, 96–97, 208–212
    ectopic beats, 91
    electrophysiology and, 96
    extrasystoles, 92–94
    harmless, 114, 114f
    invasive treatments, 113–114
    normal sinus rhythm, 90–91
    paroxysmal tachycardia, 94–97, 96f
    sudden cardiac death and, 109–110
    torsade de pointes, 110–111, 110f
    ventricular standstill, 111–112, 111f
Arteries, *See also* Coronary artery disease
    coronary, 11–12, 12f
    "hardening" of, 31
    pulmonary, 4, 4f
    "scared snake" phenomenon, 31
Asbestos, COPD and, 146
Aschoff bodies, 133, 134f
Aspirin
    as anticoagulant, 100
    for atrial fibrillation patients, 100
    discontinue before surgery, 214
    to treat myocardial infarction, 60
Asthma, 146
Atenolol, 33, 36t
Atherectomy, 173–174
Atheromas, 29, 41–43, 42f
Atria, 1, 2f
Atrial diastole, 9
Atrial ectopic tachycardia
    with AV block, 152–153
    invasive treatment of, 113
Atrial fibrillation, 97–100, 98f
    anticoagulant therapy, 99, 100
    blood clots and, 100
    causes of, 99–100
    coumadin therapy for, 214
    drug treatment for, 98–99
    invasive treatment of, 114
Atrial flutter, 100–102
    coumadin therapy for, 214
    ECG findings in, 101f
    invasive treatment of, 113

Atrial gallop, 214–215
Atrial septal defects, 123, 124f
    primum type, 123, 125f
    secundum type, 123, 124f
Atrial syncytium, 15
Atrial systole, 9, 214
Atrioventricular block, 103–106
    ECG findings in, 104–106f
    Mobitz (type II), 105–106, 107f
    types of, 104–106
    Wenckebach (type I), 104, 105f
Atrioventricular (AV) node,
    15, 17f
Atrioventricular (AV) valves, 6
Auscultation, 214–216
Autoimmune disease, 132
Autonomic nervous system, 76
AV nodal block
    atrial fibrillation and, 152
    pacemaker to treat, 151–152
AV node, 15, 17f, 80, 82, 82f
AV valves, 6

Balloon angioplasty, 173
Balloon catheter, 54f, 55f
Balloon valvuloplasty, 69, 174
Barnard, Christian, 176
Beta-blocking drugs, 33
    as cause of sick sinus syndrome, 103
    effects of, 36t
    side effects, 37t, 103
    to treat angina pectoris, 57, 58f
    to treat atrial fibrillation, 98
    to treat left heart failure, 161–162
    to treat myocardial infarction, 59
    to treat paroxysmal tachycardia, 96
Bicarbonate, 19
Bicuspid aortic valve, 120, 121f
Blood clots
    anticoagulant research and, 168
    and atrial fibrillation, 100
    pacemakers and, 154–155
Blood flow
    through the aorta, 5f
    through the heart, 2, 3f, 9–10
    through the veins and arteries, 4, 4f
Blood pressure
    control of, 59
    defined, 25
    measurement of, 25
    "normal," 25–26, 26f
    systolic/diastolic, 25
Blood pressure cuff. *See*
    Sphygmomanometer
Blood supply, 11–12
    to the brain, 29, 66, 67f
    "reserve" or collateral, 11
Blood tests, 53–54
Blue bloaters, 144–145
Bronchi, 18, 18f

Bronchioles, 18, 145
Bronchitis, 143
Brugada syndrome, 118
Bumetanide, 36t
Bundle branches, 15
    heart block and, 105–106, 106f, 151
Bundle of His, 15
Bypass grafting. *See* Coronary artery
        bypass surgery
Bypass surgery. *See* Coronary artery
        bypass surgery

Calcium, effects on ECG, 86
Calcium-blocking drugs, 35
    as cause of sick sinus syndrome, 103
    effects of, 36t
    side effects, 37t, 103, 210–211
    to treat atrial fibrillation, 98
    to treat paroxysmal tachycardia, 96
Capillaries, 4, 11
Captopril
    effects of, 36t
    side effects, 37t
Carbon dioxide, 19
Carbonic acid, 19
Cardiac arrhythmias. *See* Arrhythmias
Cardiac catheterization, 164–166,
        164f, 165f
    ejection fraction measurement, 165, 189
    need for, 166
Cardiac output, 188
Cardiac surgery, 168–177
    aortic aneurysm repair, 174–176
    bypass surgery, 62, 170–172
    for congenital heart defect repairs, 170
    history of, 168
    transplantation, 176–177
    valve replacement, 169–170, 169f
Cardiac transplantation, 176–177
    candidates for, 177
    costs of, 177
    history of, 176
    prognosis of life after, 177
Cardiocerebral resuscitation, 182
Cardiogenic shock, 49–50, 49f, 61
Cardiopulmonary resuscitation, 112–113
    new procedures for, 181–182, 183f, 184f,
        185–187
Carotid sinus syncope, 153
Carvedilol, 161
Casual coronary artery disease, 148–149
Catapress, 32, 33f, 37t
Catecholamine-blocking drugs, 32–33, 33f
    effects of, 36t
    side effects, 37t
Catecholamines, 31–32, 39
Catheter, defined, 164
Catheterization, cardiac, 164–166,
        164f, 165f
Cerebral hyperfusion, 40

Cerebrovascular accident, 28
Chorea, 124
Chronic left heart failure, 160–161
    treatment of, 160–161
Chronic obstructive pulmonary disease
        (COPD), 143–145
    smoking as cause of, 146
    treatment of, 146
Cigarette smoking
    heart disease and, 20
    relation to COPD, 146
Circumflex artery. *See* Left circumflex
        artery
Clonidine, 32, 33f
    effects of, 36t
    side effects, 37t, 103
Coarctation of the aorta, 127, 127f
    cardiac surgery repair, 170
Combined heart failure, 162
Complete heart block, 107–109
    diagnosis of, 107
    ECG findings in, 108f
    pacemakers and, 109
Congenital aortic stenosis, 120–121
    symptoms of, 120, 121
Congenital heart disease, 120–131
    advice for parents of a child with, 131
    aortic stenosis, 120–121, 121f
    cardiac surgery repairs, 170
    causes of, 120
    coarctation of the aorta, 127, 127f
    complete transposition of the great
        vessels, 129–131, 130f
    endocarditis, 131
    patent ductus arteriosus, 125, 126f
    pregnancy and, 141–142
    pulmonic valve stenosis, 128, 128f
    septal defects, 121–125
    tetralogy of Fallot, 128–129, 129f
Congestive heart failure, 27–28, 37, 66, 68
    atrial fibrillation as cause of, 97
    in pregnancy, 140, 142
    rotating tourniquets treatment, 158f
COPD (chronic obstructive pulmonary
        disease), 143–145
    smoking as cause of, 146
    treatment, 146
Copeland, Jack, 176
Cor pulmonale, 143, 156
Coronary arteries, 11–12, 12f, 62
Coronary arteriography, 53, 147
    abuses of, 167
    reasons for, 166
Coronary artery bypass surgery, 170–172
    conditions for, 62, 171
    history of, 170
    principle of, 171f
    prognosis in, 172
    risks in, 172
    technique of, 170, 172f

Coronary artery disease, 29, 41–64
  causal, 148–149
  diagnosis of, 50–55
  invasive vs. noninvasive diagnosis
    and treatment, 62–63
  mortality from, 170t
  prevention, 63, 156
  treatment of, 55–63
Coronary atheromatosis, 41–50
Coronary insufficiency, 47
Coronary "pain." *See* Angina pectoris
Coronary sinus, 11
Coronary spasm, 148
Coronary veins, 11
Cortisols, 39
Coumadin, 100
  current notes on, 213–214
  risk factors during pregnancy,
    140, 142
Crescendo angina, 47, 47f
  diagnosis of, 51–53
  heparin therapy for, 214
  treatment of, 58–59

Defibrillator, implantable, 111, 112f, 118
Delirium cordis, 97
Dependent edema, 24
Diagnostic procedures. *See*
    Echocardiography; Radioisotope
    testing
Diastole, 6, 9, 13–14, 15f
Diastolic hypertension, 26
Diazoxide, 40
Dicumarol, 168
Digitalis
  with ACE inhibitors, 162
  as cause of sick sinus syndrome, 103
  effect on ECG, 87
  for paroxysmal supraventricular
    tachycardia, 96
  pharmacology of, 209
  toxic rhythms as side effect of,
    116–117
  to treat arrhythmias, 98–99, 162
  to treat atrial fibrillation, 98–99
  to treat left heart failure, 159, 162
  vagal effect and, 79
Dihydropyridine calcium blockers, 210
Diltiazem
  effects of, 36t
  side effects, 37t
Direct dilators, 33, 34f, 36t
Disopyramide, 99, 211
Diuretics
  effects of, 36t, 158, 158f
  side effects, 37t
  to treat heart failure, 158, 160–161
  to treat hypertension, 31
Down syndrome, 120
Dyspnea, 22–23, 37, 52

ECG. See Electrocardiogram (ECG)
Echocardiography
  for ejection fraction measurement, 189
  indications for, 192–193
  M-mode display method, 190, 191f
  stress testing and, 88
  two-dimensional (2-D) method, 189, 190,
    191f, 192f, 193f
Ectopic beats, 91, 92
  atrial ectopic beats, 92, 93f, 94f
Edema
  dependent, 24
  pulmonary, 23, 24f, 27–28
Eisenmenger phenomenon, 122, 123f
Ejection fraction, 165
  defined, 188–189
  measurement of, 188–189, 189f
Electrocardiogram (ECG), 80–89
  and chamber enlargement,
    85–86
  electrode placement, 81f
  interpretation of, 80
  for myocardial infarction diagnosis, 53,
    62, 84–86
  normal vs. abnormal, 50f, 83f
  and stress testing, 50–53, 86–89
  wave names, 83
  waves of, 17f, 18, 80, 83–85
Electrophysiology, 14–18
Emphysema, 143
Enalapril
  effects of, 36t
  side effects, 37t
End arteries, 11
Endocarditis, 73–75
  acute, 74
  prevention, 75
  prophylaxis, for childbirth, 75
  prophylaxis, for dental procedures, 75
  prophylaxis, for mitral valve prolapse,
    76, 170
  risk factors for, 74, 131
  subacute, 74
  treatment of, 74–75
  vegetations, 73, 74f
Endocardium, 8
Epicardium, 8
Essential hypertension, 30–31
Ethacrynic acid
  effects of, 36t
  side effects, 27t
Exercise, for coronary disease
    prevention, 63
Exercise stress testing, 50–52, 62,
    86–89
Extrasystoles, 92–94

Favaloro, Rene, 170
Fibrillation, defined, 97
First-degree heart block, 104

Flecainide, 99, 211
Fourth heart sound,
    214–215
Furosemide
    effects of, 36t, 158, 158f
    side effects, 37t

Genetics, sudden cardiac death and,
    117–119
Great vessels of the heart, 5
    ECG findings, 130f
    transposition of, 129–131
Gruentzig, Andreas, 173
Guanabenz, effects of, 36t
Guanethidine, 32, 33f
    effects of, 36t

"Hardening" of the arteries, 31
Harvey, William, 2
Heart
    blood flow through, 2, 3f,
        9–10
    blood supply to, 11–12
    chambers of, 1, 2f
    connection to lungs, 2–5
    electrical system, 14–18
    function of, 13–20
    great vessels of, 5
    layers of, 8, 8f
    as oxygen pump, 18–20
    structure of, 1–5
    valves of, 6–7
Heart attack, 38, 40, 178–187, *See also*
        Angina pectoris; Myocardial
        infarction; Myocardial ischemia
    first aid for, 181–187
Heart block
    complete, 107–109, 108f, 151
    first-degree, 104
    Mobitz (type II), 104–106, 107f
    second-degree, 104
    sick sinus syndrome and,
        102–103
    Wenckebach (type I), 104, 105f
Heart disease, *See also* Coronary artery
        disease; Infectious heart disease
    cigarette smoking and, 20
    functional classification of,
        138–140, 139f
    infectious, 70–75
    pregnancy and, 138–142
Heart failure, 21–24
    acute left, 157–160, 178–179, 179f
    betablockers and, 161–162
    chronic left, 160–161
    combined, 162
    congestive, 27–28, 37, 66, 68
    isolated or "pure" right, 162
    left, 21–23
    right, 23–24

tourniquets for treatment of, 157–158,
        157f, 158f, 162
    treatment of, 156–163
Heart-lung machine, 168, 169f
Heart murmur, 215
Heart rhythms. *See* Arrhythmias
Heart transplantation. *See* Cardiac
        transplantation
Heart valves. *See* Valves
Heartbeat, *See also* Arrhythmias
    cycle of a, 9
    ectopic beats, 91
    origin of, 91f
Heberden, William, 43
Hemoglobin, oxygenation of, 19, 19f
Heparin, 168, 213–214
High blood pressure. *See* Hypertension
Holter, Eric, 89
Holter monitor, 89
Hydralazine, 33, 36t, 37t, 162
Hydrochlorothiazide, 37t
Hypertension
    causes of, 30–31
        linked to kidney disease, 30
        obesity, 35
        salt intake and, 30–31
    complications of, 27–30
        strokes and, 29
    defined, 25–26
    "essential," 30
    kinds or types of, 26–27
        accelerated or malignant,
            35–36
        adrenal, 39
        adrenocortical adenoma, 39
        diastolic, 26
        renal or kidney, 38–39
        systolic, 26
    in pregnancy, 138, 140
    prevention, 40
    treatment
        calcium blockers, 35
        catecholamine-blocking drugs,
            32–33
        combined therapy, 35
        direct dilators, 33, 34f, 36t
        diuretics, 31
        drug therapy, 31–35, 36t, 37t
        salt restrictions, 30–31
        spironolactone, 35
        weight loss, 35
Hypertensive crisis, 36–38
    notes for critical care personnel, 40
    treatment, 37–38
Hypertensive heart disease,
    25–40
Hypervolemic, 160

Ibutilide, 211
Imaginary spasm, 148

Infarct
    defined, 47
    post-thrombolytic, 70
Infection, pacemakers and, 154
Infectious heart disease, 70–75
Inferior vena cava, 3f, 4
Invasive diagnosis and treatment, 62–63,
        113–114
Isosorbide, 161
Isosorbide dinitrate, 57

Jenner, Edward, 43
Jervell and Lange-Nielsen syndrome, 117
Jorpes, J. Eric, 168

Kidney disease and hypertension, 30
Kidney failure, 29–30

LAD (left anterior descending) artery, 12,
        12f, 41, 62
LCA (left circumflex artery), 12, 12f, 41
Left anterior descending (LAD) artery, 12,
        12f, 41, 62
Left bundle branch, 15
Left circumflex artery (LCA or LCirc), 12,
        12f, 41
Left heart, 1
    pressure measurements, 179–180
Left heart failure, 21–23
    acute, 157–160
    treatment of, 157–160
Left main coronary artery (LMCA), 12, 12f,
        41, 62
Left ventricular end-diastolic pressure
        (LVEDP), 207–208, 212
Lidocaine, 96
    pharmacology of, 210
Likoff, William, 147
Likoff-X syndrome, 147
Link, Karl Paul, 168
Lisinopril
    effects of, 36t
    side effects, 37t
LMCA (left main coronary artery), 12, 12f,
        41, 62
Loop diuretics, 36t
Lungs, See also Pulmonary heart disease
    anatomy of, 18f
    connection to heart, 2–5
LVEDP (left ventricular end-diastolic
        pressure), 207–208, 212

Malignant hypertension, 35–36
Massaging the heart, 183f, 184f
Methyldopa, 32, 33f
    effects of, 36t
Metoprolol, 33, 36t
Mexiletine, 99, 211
Minipress, 33, 37t
Minoxidil, 33, 36t, 37t

Mitral regurgitation, 69–70, 70f, 215
Mitral stenosis, 68–69, 134, 168
    balloon valvuloplasty for, 174
Mitral valve, 6
    closed heart surgery, 168, 169f
    disorders of, 68–70
    rheumatic heart disease damage,
        69f, 134
Mitral valve prolapse, 75–76, 76f
Mobitz II heart block, 104–105
    diagnosis of, 106, 107f
    ECG findings in, 107f
    pacemaker to treat, 151
Morphine, to treat left heart failure, 159
Mouth-to-mouth resuscitation, 184f
MUGA (multiple gated acquisition) scan,
        189, 193–194, 194f
Murmurs, 215
Myocardial hypoperfusion, 40
Myocardial infarction, 44f, 47–50
    diagnosis of, 53–55, 62, 80, 84–86
    ECG findings in, 62, 84–86
    first aid for, 180
    sequence of events, 46f
    treatment of, 59–62
Myocardial ischemia, 180
Myocarditis, 72–73, 156
    diagnosis of, 73
    in pregnancy, 138
    treatment of, 73
Myocardium, 8

Nicardipine
    effects of, 36f
    side effects, 37t
Nifedipine
    contraindications, 40
    effects of, 36t
    side effects, 37t
Nitric oxide, 57
Nitroglycerin, 40, 56–57, 161
    cautions about, 212
    for right ventricular infarction, 213
Nitroprusside, 33, 36t, 37, 40, 159, 161

Obesity, 35, 63
Overventilation, 185–186
Oxygen
    and breathing centers for COPD
        patients, 145
    distribution of, 18–20
    requirements of heart muscle, 56
    to treat left heart failure, 159, 160, 161
    to treat myocardial infarction, 59
Oxyhemoglobin, 19, 19f

P wave, 80, 82f, 85, 86f, 90, 90f
Pacemakers, 150–155
    clinical evaluations, 151
    complications of, 154–155

guidelines for, 151–152
indications for, 150
Mobitz type II block, 151
normalizing, 155
referring a patient for, 153–154
technical and mechanical problems, 150, 155
temporary pacing wires, 151
to treat complete heart block, 109, 151
to treat sick sinus syndrome, 103, 152
Parasympathetic nerves, 77
Paroxysm, defined, 94
Paroxysmal atrial tachycardia (PAT), 116–117, 117f
Paroxysmal tachycardia, 94–97, 96f
drug treatment for, 96–97
Patent ductus arteriosus, 125, 126f
Penicillin, to treat rheumatic fever, 136–137
Pericardial rub, 215–216
Pericarditis, 70–71, 72f
ECG findings in, 86
Pericardium, 8
Peripartum cardiomyopathy, 141, 142
Phenoxybenzamine, 36t
Phentolamine, 36t
Phenytoin, pharmacology of, 212
Pheochromocytoma, 39
Pink puffers, 143
Post-thrombolytic infarct, 60
Potassium, effects on ECG, 86
PR interval, 82, 82f
Prazosin, 33, 37t
Preeclampsia, 140
Pregnancy
anticoagulant risk factors, 140
congenital heart defects and, 141–142
congestive heart failure in, 140, 142
heart disease and, 138–142
hypertension and, 138, 140
peripartum cardiomyopathy in, 141, 142
rheumatic carditis in, 138, 141
Preload
defined, 160
lowering, 161
Premature atrial beats, 93f, 94f, 95f
Prinzmetal angina, 46, 46f
Prinzmetal, Myron, 46
Procainamide, 97, 99, 102
pharmacology of, 209–210
Propranolol, 33, 36t
Pulmonary artery, 4, 4f
normal vs. arteriosclerosis, 122f, 123f
Pulmonary edema, 23, 24f
acute, 23
in congestive heart failure, 27–28
Pulmonary heart disease, 20, 143–146
breathing and, 145–146
COPD, 143–145

smoking as cause of, 146
Pulmonary veins, 4
Pulmonic valve, 6
Pulmonic valve stenosis, 70, 128, 128f, 130f
Purkinje fibers, 15, 17f

Q wave, 83, 84
QRS complex, 80, 83, 84, 85
width of, 82, 82f, 90f
QT intervals, 82–83, 219t
Quinidine, 97, 99, 102, 103
pharmacology of, 208–209

R wave, 83
Radioisotope testing, 88, 189, 193–194
Receptor or receiving elements, 33
Refractory period, 97
Regurgitant murmurs, 215
Regurgitation
aortic, 68, 68f
defined, 65
mitral, 69–70, 70f, 215
tricuspid, 70, 215
Renal or kidney hypertension, 38–39
Renin, 33, 34f
Reserpine, 32, 33f
effects of, 36t
side effects, 37t
Review test, 195–200
answers, 201–206
Rheumatic carditis, 134f, 141
Rheumatic fever, 65, 132
cause of, 132
course of, 135–136
diagnosis of, 135
effects on body of, 132–134, 133f
penicillin as treatment for, 136–137
Rheumatic heart disease, 69f
characteristics of, 134–135
pregnancy and, 138, 141
Right bundle branch, 15
Right coronary artery (RCA), 12, 12f, 41
Right heart, 1
pressure measurements, 179–180
Right heart failure, 23–24
Romano-Ward syndrome, 117
Rubs, 215–216

S wave, 83
SA node, 15, 16f, 17f, 80
arrhythmias of, 90–91, 91f
normal rhythms, 90, 90f
Salt intake and hypertension, 30–31
Sarcoidosis, 146
Second-degree heart block, 104
Septal defects
atrial, 123, 124f, 125f
cardiac surgery for, 170

Eisenmenger phenomenon, 122, 123f
ventricular, 121–123, 122f, 215
Septum, defined, 1
Short QT syndrome, 118
Shortness of breath. *See* Dyspnea
Sick sinus syndrome
  causes of, 103
  "false" diagnosis of, 103
  heart block and, 102–103,
    102f
  incidence of, 103
  pacemaker to treat, 103, 152
  symptoms of, 102
Silica inhalation, and COPD, 146
Sinoatrial (SA) node, 15, 16f,
  17f, 80
  arrhythmias of, 90–91, 91f
  normal rhythms, 90, 90f
Smoking. *See* Cigarette smoking
Sotalol, 99, 211
Sphygmomanometer, 25
Spironolactone, 35
  effects of, 36t
  side effects, 37t
ST segment, 83, 84–85, 84f, 85f
St. Vitus' dance, 134
Stenosis
  aortic, 65–67, 66f, 120–121, 121f
  defined, 65
  mitral, 68–69
  pulmonic, 70, 128, 128f, 130f
Stern, Shlomo, 52
"Stoppage" of the heart
  diagnosing, 180, 181f
  first aid for, 180, 181f
"Strep throat," 132
Streptococcus, group A beta-hemolytic,
  132, 133f, 136
Stress echocardiography, 88
Stress reduction, 63
Stress testing, 50–52, 62
  accuracy of test, 87
  ECG findings in, 86–89
  effects of digitalis on, 87
  scoring of, 88
  syndrome X (false-positives), 88
  variations of, 89
Stroke, 28–29
  causes of, 29, 40
  hypertensive crisis and, 38
Stroke volume, 188
Sudden cardiac death, 109–110
  genetics and, 117–119
Superior vena cava, 3f, 4
Supraventricular beats, 92, 93f, 94f
Supraventricular, defined, 96
Supraventricular tachycardia, 95,
  96–97
  drug treatment for, 96
  invasive treatment of, 113

Swan-Ganz catheter, 207–208
SWIFT (Should We Intervene Following
  Thrombolysis) study, 60
Sympathetic nerves, 32–33, 32f, 77
Syncope
  carotid sinus, 153
  without obvious cause, 153
Syndrome X, 88, 147–148
Systole, 9, 13, 14f
Systolic hypertension, 26, 31

T wave, 83, 83f, 84, 85f
Tachycardia, defined, 94
Tachycardia, wide-beat, 115, 115f
Tachycardia-bradycardia syndrome,
  102, 102f
Tachyphylaxis, 161
Tamponade, 72f
Tetralogy of Fallot, 128–129, 129f
  ECG findings, 130f
T-F-M-O treatments, 159
Thallium-201 scanning, 88
Thiazides, effects of, 36t
Thrombolytic agents, 60
Thrombus, 47
TIMI (Thrombolysis in Myocardial
  Infarction) IIa study, 60
Timolol, 36t
Torsades de pointes, 110–111, 110f
Tourniquets, for heart failure treatment,
  157–158, 157f, 158f, 162,
  178–179, 179f
Trachea, 18, 18f
Transplant surgery. *See* Cardiac
  transplantation
Tricuspid insufficiency, 154
Tricuspid regurgitation, 70, 215
Tricuspid valve, 6
  disorders of, 70, 71f
Troponin, 54
Tuberculosis, 146
  and pericarditis, 71

Vagal effect, 79
Vagus nerve, 77–79, 153
  stimulation of, 78f
Valves, 65–76
  bioprostheses, 67f, 169
  defined, 6
  disorders of, 65–70
  four types of, 6
  function of, 6, 7f, 8
  mechanical prostheses,
    169f, 170
  replacement surgery, 169–170
Valvuloplasty, 69
Vasodilators, 34f, 37t
Vegetations, 73, 74f
Veins, coronary, 11
Ventricles, 1, 2f

Ventricular beats, 94f
Ventricular complex, 80,
    82–83
Ventricular diastole, 9
Ventricular fibrillation
    ECG findings in onset of,
        48f, 109f
    sudden cardiac death and, 48,
        109–110
Ventricular function, 188
Ventricular septal defects, 121–123,
    122f, 215
Ventricular standstill, 111–112
    ECG findings and, 111f
    treatment, 111–112

Ventricular systole, 9, 13
Ventricular tachycardia, 95,
    96–97
    drug treatment for, 96
    invasive treatment of, 113
Verapamil, 36t, 37t
    side effects of, 211
Viral myocarditis, 72, 73

Weight control, hypertension and,
    35, 63
Wenckebach AV block, 104, 105f
Wide-beat tachycardia, 115
    drug treatment for, 115
    ECG findings in, 115f